Take

S

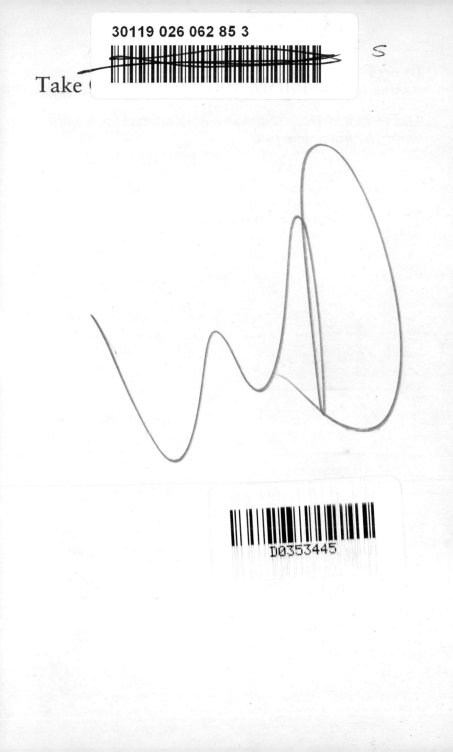

To my sisters Patricia and Susan, and all women making this transition.

And to David Hall, without whom everything would simply be much less fun.

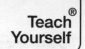

Teach®
Yourself

Take Control of
Your Menopause
Janet Wright

For UK order enquiries
130 Milton Park, Abin
Telephone: +44 (0) 12:
Lines are open 09.00–1
message answering ser
order are available at y

For USA order enquiri
Services, PO Box 545,
Telephone: 1-800-722

For Canada order enq
Ryerson Ltd, 300 Wat
Telephone: 905 430 5

Long renowned as the
with more than 50 mil
series includes over 5c
hobbies, business, com

British Library Cataloguing in Publication Data: a catalogue record
for this title is available from the British Library.

Library of Congress Catalog Card Number: on file.

First published in UK 2008 by Hodder Education,
338 Euston Road, London, NW1 3BH.

First published in US 2008 by The McGraw-Hill Companies, Inc.

This edition published 2010.

Previously published as *Teach Yourself Your Menopause*.

The **Teach Yourself** name is a registered trade mark of
Hodder Headline.

Typeset by MPS Limited, A Macmillan Company.

Printed in Great Britain for Hodder Education, an Hachette UK
Company, 338 Euston Road, London NW1 3BH, by CPI Cox &
Wyman, Reading, Berkshire RG1 8EX.

The publisher has used its best endeavours to ensure that the URLs
for external websites referred to in this book are correct and active
at the time of going to press. However, the publisher and the
author have no responsibility for the websites and can make no
guarantee that a site will remain live or that the content will remain
relevant, decent or appropriate.

Hachette UK's policy is to use papers that are natural, renewable
and recyclable products and made from wood grown in sustainable
forests. The logging and manufacturing processes are expected to
conform to the environmental regulations of the country of origin.

Impression number   10 9 8 7 6 5 4 3 2 1

Year   2014 2013 2012 2011 2010

Contents

Meet the author

Menopause may be a surprising subject for a Teach Yourself book. It's not a project you take up like learning Swedish or car mechanics. But about half the population is going to encounter it at some time. And it's ideally suited to the Teach Yourself template of practical action based on accurate and relevant information.

During perimenopause – the years leading up to menopause, when menstrual cycles end – hormones are going through changes that in some respects mirror those of puberty. However, it's easier to cope with the menopausal transition than with the angst and acne of the early teens. With maturity on their side, women can ride out perimenopausal mood swings and know that today's feelings of anxiety or despair are likely to have eased tomorrow. Unlike teenagers, they can control their angry impulses and work on practical solutions to any problems that arise.

It's just a question of getting the best information. And though there's a lot about, it's very often irrelevant or just plain wrong. Some writers feel so passionate about one aspect or another – say complementary therapies or hormone replacement therapy (HRT) – that they ignore the evidence for other options.

When I started writing about health in 1990, there wasn't much published for the everyday reader. The magazine I worked for then, *Health & Fitness*, was one of very few covering women's health issues, and its handful of staff spent a lot of time doing research and talking to experts to ensure that every word we wrote was accurate and up to date. Soon afterwards came an explosion of health coverage in women's magazines, newspapers and new publications. With the Internet, information on every conceivable topic became available at the click of a mouse.

However, these new conduits for information have also been exploited by canny publicists, manufacturers and quacks. What looks like a health news story, even in a national newspaper, may be a manufacturer's press release, or an Internet conspiracy theory, or a bright idea with no evidence to back it. On screen or in print, the wonder treatment you read about may be backed by good PR rather than genuine research. But when the unpaid or inexperienced writer doesn't know the difference, how can you? There is valuable information out there, but it can be hard to dig out from the acres of dross.

So, are we back where I started in 1990? Luckily, no – things have moved on in several areas. Back then, there had been hardly any scientific research done on complementary therapies, whereas now there's solid evidence about some. For orthodox treatments, too, we started hearing the expression 'evidence-based medicine' in the 1990s (a bit worrying for those who wondered what it had been based on before). And in among all the hoaxes and scams, the Internet now gives access to medical journals, authoritative health sites and forums for people to discuss their own experiences.

Manufacturers' studies have been revealed as often giving a misleading picture. That's not as obvious a conclusion as sceptics may think, since the studies are supposed to meet certain criteria. But bias can be created by simply not publishing those that find unfavourable results. The most believable research comes from independent studies, funded by governments or charities.

We now know a lot more about things like HRT, for example. Once seen as an elixir of youth, it lost its shine after causing numerous deaths from cancer. It was partially rehabilitated by new formulations. It is now known to offer limited benefits (though potentially useful if hot flushes are driving you mad), offset by increased health risks. It is a more nuanced and therefore more realistic picture than we ever had before.

Menopause is just one more transition in a woman's life. It's not a disease or an ordeal but, as with anything else, it's easier when you have all the knowledge you need. This book aims to provide women with accurate and unbiased information to chart a safe course.

Only got a minute?

What menopause means

Menopause, or 'the change of life', is when menstrual cycles come to an end. The time leading up to it is called 'perimenopause' though people often use the word 'menopause' to cover the whole thing. It happens because a woman is no longer producing enough reproductive hormones to become pregnant.

Most women notice the change starting gradually during their forties, as hormonal levels start to fluctuate. Other women only realize it's happening if they have difficulty conceiving. Menopause is completed when you have your last period. After that, you can no longer become pregnant.

A natural event in every woman's life, menopause happens at an average age of 51, give or take a few years. As the menstrual cycle is usually irregular by that stage, you can only identify the date in retrospect. A year after your last period it is safe to say you have finished the menopause if you're over 50; if you are younger, allow two period-free years. From then on, you no longer need to use contraception.

Most women have some symptoms of hormonal change during the few years leading up to menopause. But there are treatments or self-help remedies for all the symptoms, and most women find they don't need medical help.

5 Only got five minutes?

Symptoms of menopause

The hormonal changes taking place before menopause can cause a variety of symptoms, which may vary over a period of several years. For most women, these tend to be, at worst, uncomfortable or inconvenient rather than painful. It's useful to know what's going on, though, as some may be unexpected. Hormones also affect the brain and central nervous system, for example, so some women find themselves forgetting names or tripping over – problems that can be tackled and solved.

Levels of reproductive hormones start to decline from the mid-thirties. Few women notice any symptoms of change at that point, although they are becoming less fertile. The final period occurs, on average, at the age of 51, when hormonal changes have been going on for some 15 years. Very few women will have been troubled by symptoms for anywhere near that length of time, with many only really noticing when their periods become irregular.

Some women have markedly different symptoms at different stages of the menopausal transition. This may be because different hormonal events are taking place. It used to be thought that all menopausal symptoms were caused by a shortage of oestrogen, which is why early forms of HRT contained oestrogen alone. However, it's now known that the process is more complicated than that.

Early in the perimenopause, the symptoms may be caused by levels of progesterone falling while oestrogen remains in relative abundance. Or oestrogen levels may also be starting to drop but not evenly, perhaps fluctuating wildly, dropping from very high to still quite high. Meanwhile some of the other reproductive players, including follicle-stimulating hormone (FSH) and luteinizing hormone (LH), may be both rising and fluctuating. Testosterone production will probably be declining, though not necessarily at an even rate. As these hormones have different effects on the body and mind, the symptoms will vary according to what is happening inside.

Early perimenopausal symptoms may include heavy or painful periods, mood swings, fluid retention, migraine, insomnia and swollen or lumpy breasts. Towards the end of the menopausal transition, when oestrogen levels are falling, symptoms are more likely to include hot flushes, vaginal dryness and possibly heart palpitations.

However, there is no set route through the menopause and women's experiences vary widely. Women also vary in their physical sensitivity to hormones, so someone experiencing severe symptoms isn't necessarily undergoing dramatic hormonal changes. Conversely, a woman could have a lot going on hormonally without particularly noticing the effects. Personal history offers a clue: a woman who has had strong hormonal symptoms in the past, for example suffering the pains and emotional upheaval of premenstrual syndrome (PMS) before a period, is more likely to notice symptoms of the perimenopause. It's not about weakness or self-indulgence – it's just a physical variation.

On the other hand, many women barely notice menopause and aren't too bothered by the mild symptoms they may encounter. Even among women who have more noticeable symptoms, few are troubled enough to seek treatment, although numerous orthodox and complementary remedies are available for those who wish to try them.

10 Only got ten minutes?

What to do

Almost every symptom of perimenopause – the time leading up to the end of periods – has a number of possible remedies, whether self-help, complementary or medical. *Take Control of Your Menopause* explains these in detail, using latest research evidence on what is safe and effective.

The emotional and psychological effects of perimenopause may include sudden changes of mood, irritation, low spirits and loss of confidence. But women in their forties and fifties can learn coping strategies for these stressful symptoms, in the same way that they have learned many other skills by this time of life.

Few women seek medical treatment for these non-physical symptoms, which generally respond better to self-help methods than to drugs. Among the most effective solutions are meditation, guided relaxation and a host of stress-relief techniques. Nutritional deficiencies can have strong ill-effects on the mind, and are better addressed by healthy eating than by supplements. Herbal remedies may help: most noticeably, there is evidence in favour of St John's Wort for depression. Exhaustion also plays a role, with most women of this age probably getting less sleep than they need; some small lifestyle changes can solve the problem by setting up better sleep patterns. And focusing techniques can tackle the forgetfulness and confusion that some women encounter at this time. As for the loss of pleasure in life that sometimes strikes, there's now a whole field of academic research into happiness, so the self-help tips suggested here are backed by evidence.

Physical symptoms may include breast changes, digestive problems, dry skin and membranes, fluid retention (bloating), loss of co-ordination or balance, aches and pains, and problems in the genital and surrounding areas. Periods may become heavier, lighter or irregular before they eventually stop. But it's the vasomotor or 'faulty thermostat' symptoms – hot flushes and night sweats – that are most likely to drive a woman to seek medical help.

There are more remedies for physical than for non-physical symptoms, as this is where medical options may be helpful.

Oestrogen-only hormone replacement therapy (HRT) eases a lot of problems, but also sharply increases the risk of womb cancer, so it is only prescribed to women who have had a hysterectomy (removal of the womb). Combined HRT includes some progestogen (synthetic progesterone), which protects the womb but causes other side effects.

After years of research and controversy, it is now certain that combined HRT increases the risk of breast cancer, strokes and blood clots. HRT was once hoped to ward off the ills of old age, such as heart disease and dementia, but it hasn't proved effective in this area except for osteoporosis and bowel cancer. Indeed, if started after menopause, HRT increases the risk of heart disease.

However, HRT is the most effective treatment for severe hot flushes that don't respond to milder remedies. It also reduces the drying and weakening effects of menopause on the vagina and surrounding organs. These are the only two conditions for which it has been proved to work – though that is enough for the small number of women whose lives are disrupted by them. *Take Control of Your Menopause* goes into the pros and cons in sufficient detail to help anyone to understand the statistics and to decide whether HRT is for them. Doctors now recommend taking it only in the lowest dose that works, and for no more than two years.

Certain other drugs can be prescribed to tackle hot flushes and night sweats, but there's little evidence for their safety and effectiveness. Medical science has more to offer against period problems such as heavy bleeding, which can be controlled with various drugs including the contraceptive Pill, or by use of an intrauterine contraceptive system containing progestogen.

Although herbal remedies are popular, there is not much clear evidence to support their use, and some are dangerous. Other complementary therapies may be more helpful, and are less likely to cause harm. Many women have been helped by acupuncture, massage and breathing exercises.

The most effective way of coping with most perimenopausal symptoms is by making small lifestyle changes. Stop smoking, eat more vegetables, take regular exercise – helpful at any age, but essential during times of hormonal upheaval. You can even tailor your exercise routine to tackle specific symptoms. Add some t'ai chi if you're losing your balance easily, for example, or some dancing to combat fatigue, or swimming to reduce the discomfort of hot flushes.

Similarly, different foods have been found to combat various perimenopausal symptoms. Best-known are phytoestrogens, plant compounds found most abundantly in soy. As they are similar to oestrogen, they may work as a mild form of HRT. Many women have found a diet rich in soy foods reduces their hot flushes, although there isn't yet a lot of convincing published evidence either way. Though high-dosage supplements and novel soy-based foods are now available, phytoestrogens are best eaten in traditional forms until more is known about taking large doses. However, fears that phytoestrogens caused thyroid disease have not been backed by evidence.

In the postmenopausal period, the body is producing much less oestrogen than before. Because oestrogen nourishes the sex organs and surrounding area, women sometimes have lasting urogenital changes such as vaginal dryness, urinary incontinence and an increased vulnerability to infections such as thrush and cystitis. Sometimes these ease off as the body adapts to its new balance. Otherwise, there are numerous practical solutions including over-the-counter products, special exercises and oestrogen creams.

Only about one woman in ten is troubled enough by symptoms to seek medical help. And about the same number of women breeze through the menopausal transition without a care. In between, most women notice some symptoms, and the advice in *Take Control of Your Menopause* can help you to choose the course of action that suits you. It's not meant as a substitute for medical advice, though, so always see your doctor if you notice a new symptom or have any other health concern.

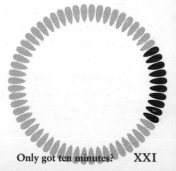

1

An introduction to the menopause

This chapter answers some frequently asked questions about the menopause.

You will learn:
- *what the menopause is and what it isn't*
- *why it's useful to understand it*
- *how to relieve symptoms, if you have any.*

Ten common questions

Q. *I'm having hot flushes. What should I do?*
A. This is the classic sign of menopausal changes, and the one most effectively relieved by HRT. See the sections on hot flushes in Chapters 9–13 for how to beat the heat.

Q. *I haven't had a period for six months. Is this the menopause?*
A. If you're over 45 and have had some signs such as hot flushes or irregular periods, or if you're over 50 (with or without symptoms), you probably have started the menopausal transition. If you're under 45, it may be an early menopause or it may have another cause, so you should consult your doctor.

Q. *How do I know I've been through the menopause?*

A. When you've had a year without periods if you're over 50, or two years if you're under 50, you can look back to the date of your final period and know that was the menopause. Many women still have symptoms for a few years after the final bleed, but they are officially 'postmenopausal'. You don't have real periods when you're on the Pill, but you may notice menopausal symptoms on the progestogen-only Pill (POP). It's harder to tell if you're taking the combined Pill, but you are recommended to stop this at 50 anyway.

Q. *How soon is it safe to stop using contraception?*

A. If you're over 50, keep using contraception until you've been a year without periods. If you're under 50, allow two period-free years. See Chapter 6 on contraception and fertility to find out what's most appropriate for you now.

Q. *My mother went through the menopause before she was 40. Does that mean I'm likely to do the same?*

A. Possibly. Premature menopause does sometimes run in families, but it's more often linked with illness or things that happened to you in childhood or before birth. See Chapter 14 on early and premature menopause.

Q. *I'm in my thirties and still hope to have children. How long can I put if off?*

A. The average woman's fertility starts a steep decline in her late thirties, when changes leading up to the menopause begin. Unfortunately there isn't a foolproof test to show you if you are 'average', as the available hormone tests can be misleading.

Q. *I'm in my mid-forties, just starting to notice signs of the menopause. Is it worth taking HRT to prevent symptoms?*

A. It's better to wait and see if you have symptoms before taking HRT. Most women find they don't need it or it doesn't suit them and HRT is only helpful for some symptoms anyway – mainly the hot flushes, night sweats and vaginal dryness. See Chapter 8 on HRT for more details.

Q. I'm considering taking HRT. What are the risks?

A. They vary a lot depending on your age, health, medical history and even genetics. In particular, the increased risk of cancer is small but significant. Unless you are suffering badly from hot flushes and night sweats, doctors now do not recommend taking HRT. If you are having trouble with those symptoms, see Chapter 8 on HRT to help you make an informed choice. To understand the research in more depth, see the Appendix.

Q. I've passed the menopause but am still suffering from fatigue and aching limbs. Should I try HRT?

A. Most studies that show the harmful effects of HRT have been carried out on women using it after the menopause, so this is not a good time to start. Also, HRT hasn't been proved effective against your symptoms. These are more likely to respond to lifestyle changes, especially exercise. See Chapters 11 and 13 on lifestyle and fitness for more information.

Q. Help, I'm piling on weight! Is this unavoidable during the menopause?

A. It's very common, and hormonal changes play a major role (see Chapter 2). You do have to work at counteracting weight gain at this time of life, but it can be done. See the chapters on nutrition and exercise for more information.

What is the menopause?

Officially, the menopause is the day your final period stops – the average age is 51. After the menopause, you can no longer become pregnant unless in exceptional circumstances. However, you can't be certain you've passed the menopause until a year has gone by without menstruation, or two years if you're under 50. Until then, there's always the chance you may just be having a very long gap between periods.

The menopause has some other meanings too. It is also:

▶ *a word widely used to mean the few years surrounding that final period, when you may experience some symptoms of hormonal change.*

▶ *a time when hormones settle into a different balance (more about that later). The body's production of oestrogen – the best-known female hormone – declines from the high levels it has maintained since puberty. Levels of progesterone and other hormones also change.*

▶ *a sentry. Your risk of certain health conditions increases with age. Men are often taken by surprise, for example, when a heart attack strikes in their fifties even though they still feel 35. These problems can't creep up on women in the same way: the menopause is an unmistakeable sign of change. And as this book will show, many weapons and tactics are available to combat health problems.*

▶ *a transition. The hormonal changes that characterize the menopause last for a few years at most. Afterwards, the body settles into a renewed stability.*

WHAT IS IT NOT?

The menopause gets a lot of bad press, often from companies with a 'treatment' to sell. In reality, it's not the dispiriting event many women expect.

▶ *It's not an ordeal. Very few women suffer serious long-term symptoms of the menopause. Most women have a small number of symptoms, some of which occur infrequently. Roughly one in five has severe symptoms, and even then the most common are uncomfortable but harmless hot flushes. At the other end of the scale, many women barely notice their menopause at all.*

▶ *It's not the end of femininity. It is, however, the end of periods, premenstrual syndrome (PMS), contraception and pregnancy scares. Freed from those, many women find their sex life is reinvigorated.*

▶ *It's not a one-way ticket to ill-health and decrepitude. The menopause actually improves the health of many women.*

More than a third of young women are short of iron, for example, as this essential mineral is carried in the blood and lost during monthly periods; a lack of iron causes exhaustion and can lead to the life-threatening condition anaemia. The menopause ends this regular loss of iron. For those women who suffered from long-standing gynaecological problems such as fibroids and endometriosis, the menopause brings nothing but relief. The action you take to manage menopausal symptoms (if you have any) can put your health on a sound footing for the future. The foods that may ease hot flushes, for example, also reduce the risk of conditions such as osteoporosis and heart disease in later life.

▶ It's not a pit of depression. Researchers have discovered that women are, on average, less likely to suffer from depression after the menopause than before. And the despair and mood swings of PMS disappear for good.

▶ It's not a time when you really ought to slow down. Numerous studies have shown that exercise can have even greater benefits during and after the menopause than before. You may well have more energy for exercise: the menopause is revitalizing to the many women who were weakened by their monthly blood loss.

▶ It's not the beginning of the end. The average woman in a developed country can look forward to nearly three more decades of life after the menopause. Perhaps surprisingly, given the pessimistic concerns expressed by politicians and the media, statistics show that most of this time will be spent able-bodied and in good health.

Glad to be free of blood and pain

'It is great not to have periods and have to spend money on all the gear,' says Ros, a charity coordinator. 'Having a young daughter means I regularly witness the impact of premenstrual tension and pain and loss of blood that periods can cause, and I am so glad to be free of it all.'

What is the perimenopause?

The perimenopause literally means 'around the time when periods stop.' But it is commonly used to refer to the years when hormone levels start changing, before periods stop altogether. The perimenopause is the early part of the stage in life popularly known as 'the menopause'. This book uses the term to refer to the time prior to periods stopping.

The word 'postmenopausal' is occasionally used to describe the rest of a woman's life, but that's a bit like calling your twenties and thirties 'post-puberty'. This book uses 'postmenopause' for the few years after periods stop, until the body has adjusted to all menopausal hormonal changes.

While many of the symptoms of the perimenopause and postmenopause are similar, the hormone picture for each stage can be very different and may require different treatment. During the early years of the perimenopause, for example, progesterone levels may be lower than usual, while oestrogen remains high. Taking remedies suitable for a later stage could be harmful. Knowing what stage you've reached allows you to take action that is both effective and safe.

Insight

As you approach the age of menopause, your body's production of reproductive hormones changes, mainly producing less than before. When the level of oestrogen drops below a certain point, your menstrual cycles stop.

Why do I need to know this information?

The menopause is as natural a stage in life as puberty, when the reproductive system starts getting into gear for future pregnancy and childbirth. But like that earlier transition, the menopause is marked by internal changes that can cause some upheaval. It's not the menopause that's being treated, but these sometimes disruptive symptoms such as hot flushes – a wave of intense heat that's caused by a sudden fluctuation in hormone production.

If any of these symptoms becomes enough of a nuisance to warrant treatment, it's useful to know what's causing them. For example, symptoms that start late in the menopause are likely to stem from a drop in oestrogen production. The most commonly used remedies for symptoms at any time during the menopause aim to replace oestrogen. However, symptoms early in the perimenopause may be caused by hormonal fluctuations, and oestrogen levels may be high in relation to progesterone. Therefore, adding more oestrogen could make the problem worse.

The reproductive hormones, including oestrogen and progesterone, can have both good and bad effects on the body. Oestrogen, for example, makes certain cancers grow faster. But they may also protect against conditions such as osteoporosis and coronary heart disease. Knowing that this protection is dwindling gives you a chance to compensate by making lifestyle changes.

Recognizing the early signs of menopause gives you a chance to take action. You may be able to delay the process or you may choose to go with it but be ready to deal with symptoms if and when they arise.

What if the menopause happens sooner than expected?

For some women, the menopause comes earlier than they expect. This may be because of lifestyle factors such as smoking or exposure to harmful chemicals. It may be a side effect of medical treatment such as chemotherapy for cancer, or the result of an operation such as a hysterectomy. Or it may stem from reasons beyond anyone's control such as genetics or a past illness.

Early menopause isn't necessarily a problem, unless you were still planning to have children. If you have had gynaecological problems, you may welcome it. But it does mean that your body has lost some of the protection conferred by the reproductive hormones, for example in keeping bones strong.

For this reason, you're more likely to be prescribed hormone replacement therapy (HRT) than if you reached menopause later. See Chapter 14 on early and premature menopause for more information.

If you're in your late thirties and hoping to have children, it's useful to know the signs of declining fertility.

Top tip

On the contraception/fertility front, don't leave things to chance unless you're very relaxed about having a baby in your forties or fifties. You can still get pregnant when you haven't had a period for months. But you can't rely on this if you want a baby.

What are the symptoms of the menopause?

Changing levels of reproductive hormones at this time can cause a variety of symptoms. Some, such as hot flushes, are well known, but others may take you by surprise because they don't seem connected with female hormones.

Symptoms may include anxiety, breast lumpiness, breast pain, clumsiness, constipation, depression, dry skin, fatigue, fluid retention (bloating), forgetfulness, gall bladder problems, headaches, heart palpitations, heavy bleeding, insomnia, irregular periods, joint pains, loss of balance, loss of libido, mental fuzziness, mood swings, night sweats, painful periods, thrush, urinary incontinence, urinary infections, vaginal dryness and weight gain. All of these symptoms are connected with changes in hormone levels, some of which affect the brain and central nervous system.

It looks like a daunting list, but remember that most women will only have a few of these symptoms, often mildly and infrequently. Indeed, many women will say they haven't had any symptoms, then rack their brains and remember that their periods became heavy and irregular before the menopause, or that they had a few hot flushes.

A list of the ill effects of pregnancy or the menstrual cycle would look just as overwhelming, until you remember that no one suffers all of them, and most women have few or minor problems.

Some of the symptoms are surprising. You wouldn't think, for example, that the menopause could make you trip over, weaken internal muscles or change the functioning of your gall bladder. That's why it's useful to know what's going on. You're not falling apart, mentally or physically. You're just going through a period of readjustment that can affect your whole body, including the brain.

Insight

It is estimated that ten per cent of women have no menopausal problems and about ten per cent have symptoms that bother them enough to seek treatment. Most women go through menopause with little or no trouble, using lifestyle changes to ease any problems that occur.

How long are the symptoms likely to last?

Most of the best-known menopausal symptoms are caused by the erratic fluctuations of hormones that are going through a major shift. Once they've settled down, these symptoms stop because your hormones have reached a new balance.

Short-term symptoms include:

▶ *the faulty thermostat: flushes, night sweats, rapid changes from cold to hot*

- *brain and nerve symptoms such as forgetfulness, mental fuzziness and clumsiness*
- *emotional symptoms such as weepiness, mood swings and anxiety*
- *all symptoms connected with the menstrual cycle, such as monthly fluid retention and PMS.*

Symptoms may last anything from a few months to eight or ten years – though it would be unusual to have seriously disruptive symptoms lasting that long. If the problem doesn't wear off by itself, most women can find a solution that will at least reduce its effects.

Some of the changes, though, are caused by the drop in production of hormones (especially oestrogen), rather than by fluctuations or by the changing ratio of one to another. So those changes will continue when hormone production has settled at this lower level.

Lasting changes may include:

- *dryness, which can lead to skin ageing, vaginal dryness, thrush and urinary infections*
- *loss of libido*
- *bladder weakness*
- *weight gain that's hard to shift, especially round the middle.*

Luckily, all of these symptoms can be dealt with, mainly by using simple remedies and lifestyle changes.

Top tip

Never presume that a new symptom is just a sign of your age. Get it checked by your doctor, as it could be caused by an illness that needs treating. Several chronic conditions become more common during this time of life, including diabetes and thyroid disease. They can be well controlled if picked up early.

What else could it be?

At this time of life, women often put any health problems down to the menopause. It's true that hormonal changes can have some unexpected effects, such as joint pains or loss of balance. But don't take this for granted – they could be caused by something else. As with any other change in your health, you should let your doctor know and get it checked out.

Most conditions are easier to treat if they're diagnosed early, when there's a good chance of keeping them under control. Joint pains, for example, might be an early sign of arthritis. A number of different neurological conditions could make you fall over – or it could just mean you're getting rather unfit and need to build up your leg muscles.

It's not just the unexpected signs, either. Some of the most common effects of the menopause could actually be signs of health conditions that need to be treated.

It's a myth, for example, that female non-smokers don't develop coronary artery disease before the menopause. Oestrogen does provide some protection from heart disease, but it's not infallible. If you're tired and breathless, at whatever age, do go to your doctor – and don't be fobbed off with 'it's just your age'.

The same goes for mood swings – famous symptoms of PMS and the menopause. They could also be a sign of other conditions, such as diabetes. How do you tell the difference? You don't – a blood test does. Even the most obvious sign of menopause, the loss of periods, can be caused by a number of other hormonal conditions. So don't take it for granted that any change is caused by the menopause.

Tell your GP about any new symptoms so that you can find out what's causing them. You can then be sure that the action you're taking to treat them is appropriate.

What can I do about it?

This book is about getting through the menopause with as little inconvenience as possible. For some women, it won't be an issue as their hormones change gear so smoothly that they barely notice the menopause, and they simply get on with their lives. For them, the information in this book is preventive and can ensure that later life continues on this healthy route.

Women who have some symptoms can find out more about their significance in the next few chapters. If it's a minor problem, just knowing its cause and effects may be enough. If it's something that bothers you, there are now numerous solutions at hand.

Some people have strong feelings about using only natural therapies. Others are equally determined to seek the best that twenty-first century medical science has to offer. If you're pragmatic, and prepared to try anything safe that might help, you increase your chances of finding a solution. The later chapters will set out the numerous options now available in orthodox and complementary therapies. Each of them will include the most reliable available evidence about their efficacy and safety.

Self-help techniques are among the most tried and tested solutions to hormone-related problems. Breathing exercises, for example, may soothe a hot flush that's already started, and aerobic exercise has been shown to reduce the likelihood of having one.

As with other choices, some people love trying new techniques, while others can't face fitting yet another task into their schedule. But self-help has something extra to offer: unlike most therapies it's almost guaranteed safe, has no side effects, costs little or nothing and is totally under your control.

There's something for everyone who is prepared to spend a little time on their own wellbeing. For more information, see Chapters 10–13 on complementary approaches, lifestyle, nutrition and fitness.

Can we trust HRT and other remedies?

Numerous studies have linked HRT with an increased risk of certain cancers and other diseases. But the picture isn't as clear as it may seem. Some studies suggest that it's only long-term use that's a problem, while others disagree on what age group is most affected. This is explained in detail in Chapter 8 on HRT.

Knowledge about medical and complementary therapies is changing fast, as both doctors and consumers demand evidence-based medicine. New drugs and processes have to undergo intensive scrutiny before patients get near them. Hundreds of studies are conducted on existing medicines to see if they can be used in different ways, or if their long-term use reveals any unexpected effects. Herbal medicines, too, are becoming tightly controlled and studied. Research into other complementary therapies has also taken off since the early 1990s.

All the information is building up a complex picture of drugs that transform some people's lives, but leave others worse off than before. Year by year, we find out more about who will benefit, and why. As complementary therapies come under the microscope, they too are revealing long-held secrets – not always in their favour.

Digging out the truth is difficult. One confusing point is that often one study will come up with results that seem to contradict another. Sometimes this is because one of the studies was based on wrong information or badly carried out. Sometimes both sets of results are valid, and what the press reported as a contradiction stems from slightly different circumstances producing different results. Sometimes the reason is less clear. And, as prestigious medical journals have recently reported, sometimes the manufacturers hide bad news or put an excessively positive slant on a study that might have shown their product in a bad light.

With complementary therapies, the difficulty is that there's still only a small body of reliable evidence. Manufacturers may be certain they have a good product, but the sort of trials that drugs go through are prohibitively expensive for a small company making herbal remedies.

On top of that is the problem of statistics. They are much more complicated than they appear at first sight. What looks like a major breakthrough often turns out to be a very small improvement. In the same way, what seems like an unacceptable side effect may affect hardly anyone. Reports of a 50 per cent increase in a rare form of cancer, for example, sound outrageous. But when you read the figures, it could just mean that three women get it in a year instead of two.

If you have a serious health condition, you have to weigh up any ill effects of treatment against the suffering you're going through now. If what you've got is not a life-threatening condition, but the treatment might cause cancer, it would need to make you feel very much better to be worth even a small risk of dying. You also have to weigh up any side effects against the benefits.

The only risk-free way of dealing with symptoms is to take no remedies at all. That's what most women with only minor or infrequent problems do. Some women who do try remedies are pleased with the results; others decide that HRT and other drugs don't do enough good to outweigh the side effects, let alone the long-term health risks. But a few get so desperate that they wouldn't care what the risk was of developing cancer some time in the future. Estimation of that risk keeps varying with every new study that's published.

If you are bothered by symptoms, why not read Chapters 11–13 on lifestyle, nutrition and fitness first to see if you can solve them without needing to take remedies? This self-help information is also valuable as a back-up if you do decide to use the treatments detailed in Chapters 8–10 on HRT, other medical help and complementary approaches.

Why does the menopause get such a bad press?

The menopause is very rarely as disruptive as you might think from reading some accounts. Most of the women who spoke of their experiences for this book commented on how little it affected them – often to their surprise!

Along with hot flushes, the most notorious symptom of the menopause is emotional upheaval. Yet emotional problems are partly a reaction to widespread prejudices about this time of life. It's not surprising that some women dread this time when it's widely described in such negative terms. On television and in novels, menopausal women are portrayed as irrational shrews in the grip of uncontrollable mood swings. The knowledge that this is fiction doesn't affect the stereotype.

It's like PMS: most women experience the occasional mood swing before a period, and a very few have PMS badly enough to disrupt their lives. But the stereotype persists of women being at the mercy of their emotions during the last few days of their menstrual cycle.

In reality, hormonal changes – whether before a period or during the menopause – can affect a woman's moods and emotions, but they don't take over her life. The menopause happens at a time when many women are coping with other changes: children growing up and leaving home; parents needing care or dying; work responsibilities changing, often with a loss of status as younger people come to power. Chapter 4 on mind and mood gives some practical advice on separating external problems from hormonal effects and dealing with both.

Although the emotional effects of the menopause are exaggerated, the effects on the brain and nervous system are hardly ever mentioned. And yet these are among the most frightening symptoms if you're not expecting them.

Fit, active women suddenly find themselves stumbling over kerbs or dropping plates. Many women suffer a loss of self-confidence when this happens, and some fear they're showing the first signs of degenerative disease. It's a relief to know that clumsiness and loss of balance are physical effects of hormonal changes on nerves and muscles – and that this is temporary. Forgetfulness and difficulty in concentrating are also quite common. This can be frightening, and deeply disorienting.

As with any other change in your health, you should check with your GP, but these side effects of hormonal upheaval usually wear off by themselves. (Some women will remember feeling this way when they were pregnant.) Chapters 4 and 13 on mind and mood and on fitness could help in the meantime. Simple exercises can improve your balance, while knowing what's happening (and that it is temporary) keeps it in perspective.

A time of reflection

'I think the time is one of reflection rather than physical difficulties, at least for me,' says Christine, an academic in her fifties. 'Apart from the obligation to watch my weight and blood pressure – I have a family history of cardiovascular problems – I have been trouble-free.

'There was the visit to the doctor to check it out. "Yes," he said. "This is it." I was about 48 by then and the periods were becoming intermittent. "Women usually follow their mothers," he continued. "Ask her what you can expect." My mother was mildly informative. "The periods just petered out," she said. "I had a few hot flushes and that was about it." And so it happened for me.'

Why do women have a menopause?

If our ancestors hadn't gone through the menopause, we might not be here now! It equips women for an essential part of their life cycle that, in earlier times, could have made the difference to a tribe's survival. We don't know the cause for certain, but this is a theory that makes sense.

Humans aren't the only species that has a menopause, but we are in a small minority. Most female animals continue to ovulate until they die.

But childbearing puts a strain on even a young, fit woman's body, let alone one that has already been through a dozen pregnancies. Childbirth used to be a common cause of maternal death; it still is in much of the developing world. Babies born to dying women had very little chance of survival themselves, and the loss of their mother put her older children's lives at risk too.

Effective contraception has been widely available for less than 100 years. Through most of history, only the menopause could put an end to evermore-tiring pregnancies. This is what gives rise to the 'grandmother hypothesis' – the idea that menopause is valuable to the human race.

Among our long-ago ancestors, as soon as a woman stopped having babies, her existing children's chances of survival increased sharply. She was also able to help her daughters through their own pregnancies, and even provide for her grandchildren if her daughters died. In a harsh and hungry world, the menopause increased her own, her children's and her grandchildren's chances of survival.

Random chance throws up all kinds of mutations, so the hypothesis is that some women just happened to be born with ovaries that would fail in middle age. Unlike, say, heart failure, this turned out to be not only harmless but an advantage. These women may have had fewer babies, but more of their children survived.

This meant that, in each generation, more and more girls inheriting this useful characteristic lived to bring up families of their own. They passed it down to their own numerous descendants, and eventually to the entire human race.

This is just a hypothesis: there's no way of proving what actually happened. But scientists now believe that the human race has been through at least one period when numbers dwindled close to the point of extinction. Who knows, a group of experienced and active older women may have tipped the balance in favour of their tribe's survival.

Insight

Did menopause really help the human race survive? We can't be sure. But it certainly saved countless women from death in middle-aged childbirth – and still does, for those without access to reliable contraception.

The information in this book is not a replacement for qualified medical advice. Please consult your doctor if you have any symptoms that cause you concern, and before making any changes in medication (including alternative/complementary remedies).

A MESSAGE TO FRIENDS AND FAMILY

The menopause is a time of hormonal changes that have wide-reaching effects on all the body's systems. Some women barely notice the effects and aren't at all bothered by them. Others go through pain and ill-health while their hormones are struggling to find a new balance. Sleeplessness and digestive problems are common at this time, making everything else harder to cope with.

Many women going through the menopause have times when they feel sick, stressed or exhausted. It's not all in their minds. If a woman in your life is working through this transition, show a bit of understanding. She's dealing with major physical changes, including the temporary effects of hormonal fluctuations on the brain. Tiredness is part of this, so give her a hand when she needs it. Sometimes, the best thing anyone can do is the washing-up.

Summary

The menopause is a natural stage in life. But, like other natural events such as periods or childbirth, it can cause problems, and you don't have to put up with them. Problems may be emotional or sexual as well as physical, and some may be unexpected. Most women have quite minor symptoms, some have none at all and some have serious difficulties that can be alleviated with the right treatments. Sometimes the menopause comes early, and if you're still planning to have children, you need to be aware of signs that your fertility is waning. This book will try to explain everything you want to know and set out all the options, on the basis of the most reliable evidence.

Action plan: knowledge is power

1 *If you're experiencing some symptoms, first find out what's causing them. They may not be related to your hormones, but could be a sign of a health condition that needs attention.*
2 *If symptoms are hormonal, you may need tests done to identify what stage of the perimenopause you're in, to help you make the best choice about treatments. Later chapters will explain how to do this, and give all the different options for medical, complementary and self-help solutions.*
3 *Don't feel you have to make one choice and stick to it. Be open to trying a pick-and-mix selection of medical and complementary therapies to find what suits you best at various stages.*
4 *Self-help strategies can help in relieving many symptoms of the menopause. So be prepared to make a few small but healthy changes.*
5 *When it gets you down, remember that the menopause doesn't last long, isn't fatal, and puts an end to PMS for good.*

10 THINGS TO REMEMBER

1 Menopause means the time when your menstrual periods stop permanently.

2 It usually happens naturally, at an average age of 51.

3 Menopause is sometimes brought on early, by illness, medical treatment or other reasons.

4 After menopause you can no longer become pregnant naturally.

5 Perimenopause is the time leading up to menopause, when hormonal levels are changing.

6 It can cause a range of symptoms, both physical and non-physical.

7 It happens at a time when women are often busy with many responsibilities, so what seems to be a hormonal symptom may just stem from exhaustion.

8 Most symptoms wear off by themselves in time.

9 A small minority of women has symptoms serious enough to seek treatment.

10 Menopause puts an end to all period-related problems. It can also relieve a number of health conditions including anaemia and migraine.

2

The hormone story

In this chapter you will learn:
- *how production of reproductive hormones changes as you go through menopause*
- *if you need to discover your hormonal status*
- *what other hormones are important*
- *why hormones may affect you in surprising ways.*

This chapter starts with an explanation of the endocrine (hormone) system – what hormones are and how they affect our lives, including the menopause. This will help you to understand more about how the menopause happens. This, in turn, will make it clearer what is a short-term symptom caused by hormonal levels fluctuating in relation to each other, and what is likely to be a longer-term result of a drop in hormone production. This is particularly useful if you're considering hormone replacement therapy (HRT) or other medical treatments.

Hormones: the background

Hormones are chemicals that carry messages from one part of the body to another. They are produced in various organs (including the brain) and travel in the bloodstream.

The body produces many hormones for different purposes. Mainly, they make sure everything in our bodies stays as it is unless it needs to change for some reason. Some hormones keep our fluid levels at a steady 70 per cent, for example. Others ensure there's just the right amount of glucose in the blood to supply all our cells with energy. Too much will cause infections and eventually death, too little and you're starving.

Still other hormones affect our emotions, help to digest food, wake us and send us to sleep at the right time, and carry out many other tasks that keep us functioning normally. In emergencies, the adrenal glands produce the hormone adrenaline, which tells the heart to beat faster and the liver to release glucose for quick energy.

Insight
Most hormones are made in the endocrine glands, which are attached to various organs. Small amounts can also be made outside these glands. Oestrogen, for example, may also be produced in the breasts and other fatty tissue.

Imbalances and deficiencies

Hormonal imbalances can cause a host of problems including menstrual disorders, depression, weight gain, acne, permanently bad hair or a total loss of sex drive. They often leave you feeling constantly tired for no good reason. Rather than an overnight change, they tend to creep up on you gradually, so you forget how much better you could feel. Sometimes hormonal problems are caused by other illnesses (especially tumours), or are the side effects of medicines. Hormonal problems may also run in families.

Imbalances can lead to serious illness. Growth hormone, for example, helps build and repair muscles. Most of it is produced by the pituitary gland at night, so if your sleep is disturbed, you often wake feeling tired and achy. Some experts suspect a link with myalgic encephalomyelitis (ME) and fibromyalgia – sufferers of both conditions often sleep badly and have a lot of muscle pain. Unlike everyday insomniacs, sufferers tend to miss out on the particular phase of deep sleep when most growth hormone is produced. So their conditions may be worsened by not producing enough of it.

The best-known hormone-deficiency disease is diabetes. It's caused by a lack of insulin, which regulates the amount of glucose (sugar) in the blood. Blood glucose levels rise dangerously, damaging the organs if it's not caught in time. You may find yourself constantly running to the loo because your body is producing gallons of urine to try to flush the excess glucose out. This makes you terribly thirsty, and the high sugar levels in your body also cause infections like thrush. With prompt treatment, though, diabetes can be kept safely under control.

Reproductive hormones

The hormones people usually mean, when they think about their hormones, are the reproductive ones. Like almost everything in the stupendously complex organism of our bodies, they play many roles, large and small, in the body's functioning. They even affect our minds by influencing the brain's production of chemicals called neurotransmitters. These chemicals affect our emotions and cognitive functions such as memory and decision-making. But the reproductive hormones' major role is to regulate our menstrual cycles and pregnancies.

Throughout this book, most references to 'hormones' will mean reproductive hormones.

The two best-known reproductive hormones are oestrogen and progesterone. Progesterone is the main hormone that balances oestrogen, and when everything is functioning smoothly this works in a stately rhythm like the tides. During times of transition, such as the menopause, this balance breaks down for a while.

Levels of reproductive hormones change and fluctuate throughout our lives. The most noticeable changes occur:

- ▶ *during puberty, when we start having periods*
- ▶ *throughout pregnancy and for some time after childbirth*
- ▶ *during the few years before and after our final period – the menopause.*

However, for about 40 years after puberty, we are also producing different levels of hormones during every menstrual cycle (see below). In an ideal world, the whole system would work smoothly. But many factors, from anxiety to the food we eat, can affect hormone production enough to throw it off balance. And some women are just more sensitive than others to hormonal changes. Many women experience mood swings, tiredness or food cravings just before a period is due. Some women have it badly enough to be diagnosed with premenstrual syndrome (PMS).

So most women will have already experienced some kind of hormonal upheaval before the menopause. The end of the reproductive years is just another transition. The body's production of these hormones naturally slows down as we get older. By their late fifties, most women will have stopped having periods and hormone production will be stabilizing at a new and lower level.

SOME OF THE MAIN PLAYERS IN REPRODUCTION

- ▶ *Oestrogen (or 'estrogen' in the USA) plays the biggest role in our reproductive life. It's sometimes referred to as 'oestrogens' because it comes in three slightly different forms: oestrone, oestradiol and oestriol (or estrone, estradiol and estriol, or E1, E2 and E3). It is mainly produced in the ovaries and helps prepare for pregnancy. But this fertility has a downside too: oestrogen helps cancers grow in the breast and womb. Oestrogen isn't only the star of the reproductive show; its many other actions include preventing bone loss, counteracting inflammation and healing wounds by encouraging blood to clot. Its psychological effects are enlivening and upbeat,* but when it gets out of balance with other hormones it can make you feel irritated or angry.

▶ Progesterone is released after ovulation and starts preparing the womb lining for a pregnancy. If a fertilized egg is implanted, progesterone works throughout the pregnancy to keep it safe. But if not, the womb lining is sloughed off, a period starts and the menstrual cycle begins again. In addition to its physical functions, progesterone has a calming effect that limits oestrogen's hyperactive tendencies. Therefore, of course, too much progesterone could make you feel depressed. Progesterone can be converted into other hormones when they're needed, including oestrogen.

▶ Testosterone and other androgens (or 'male hormones') aren't just for men: they also play many roles in women's bodies. In the right amounts, testosterone provides energy and sex drive, but in excess it can cause aggression. Production spikes at around the time of ovulation, increasing our sex drive at the optimal time for conception, and shortly before a period is due, when it can fuel PMS. Levels fall towards the end of the menopausal transition, when periods stop.

▶ Dehydroepiandrosterone, or DHEA, is made in the adrenal glands from cholesterol. This is the precursor to several sex hormones.

▶ Follicle-stimulating hormone (FSH) helps the ovaries bring an egg to maturity each month. It is only produced in large quantities when there isn't much oestrogen in the body. A high FSH level is normal during the first week of the menstrual cycle, and after the menopause. At other times, in women who are still having periods, it could mean a lack of oestrogen – a possible warning of premature menopause. Low FSH levels can cause your periods to stop.

▶ Luteinizing hormone (LH) causes the ovary to release the egg when it is ready to be fertilized. Before the menopause, LH levels are usually low except around the time of ovulation. As with low FSH, high LH levels in woman who are still menstruating can be a warning of menopausal changes.

▶ Gonadotrophin-releasing hormone (GnRH) controls production of FSH and LH.

The menstrual cycle

We're born with hundreds of thousands of minuscule eggs in tiny sacs called follicles, inside the ovaries. When we reach puberty, these start ripening, and we begin the menstrual cycles that will continue until the menopause.

Day 1 is the first day of bleeding. It follows a drop in production of both progesterone and oestrogen, which triggers the uterus to slough off its lining as conception has not taken place. Oestrogen levels are low, which allows the production of FSH to start rising.

By the end of the first week, FHS has stimulated one of the follicles to grow, and the follicle now starts producing a lot of oestrogen. This in turn reduces FSH levels during the second week, while oestrogen levels peak during the second and third weeks.

About day 14 of a 28-day cycle, LH levels rise sharply, for just long enough to trigger ovulation: the follicle expels the egg into the fallopian tube on its way to the womb. Testosterone production also jumps at this time.

The collapsed follicle (called the corpus luteum) then produces progesterone during weeks three and four, to prepare the womb for a pregnancy. If the egg has not been fertilized, the cycle ends with another burst of testosterone and a steep fall in levels of oestrogen and progesterone. This causes the womb to shed its unused lining, and the cycle starts again.

Top tip

If you're looking up information on the Internet, remember that US spellings are widely used. For example, words that start with 'oest', as in oestrogen, will start with 'est', as in 'estrogen'. Gonadotrophin is spelled 'gonadotropin'. Hot flushes are 'hot flashes'.

What happens to hormones during the menopause?

It used to be thought that menopausal symptoms were simply the result of the body's production of oestrogen slowing down to a halt. That's why the first forms of hormone replacement therapy (HRT) were oestrogen-only.

It's now recognized that our systems are a lot more complex than that. Lack of oestrogen is what will eventually stop your periods, but levels of progesterone and other hormones are also changing in ways that can have noticeable effects.

As the menopause approaches, the menstrual cycle's beautifully orchestrated rhythm starts to falter. Progesterone levels fall. Oestrogen levels may also fall, or they may remain high but fluctuate with sharp drops and peaks. FSH levels may also fluctuate, but are usually quite high; the same may happen with LH.

These hormonal fluctuations are the cause of most menopausal symptoms. All the body's systems are programmed to keep everything in balance, and it makes huge efforts to compensate when something changes. But if these efforts don't succeed, its next step is to adapt to the new circumstances, which it does amazingly well.

After your periods have stopped, oestrogen levels continue to fall for a while. That's why some symptoms may continue for a year or two after the menopause. But within a few years, the hormones settle into their new routine. Oestrogen and progesterone levels are low, FSH and LH are higher than before.

Insight

Most menopausal symptoms disappear soon after your periods stop. Those that are caused by fluctuating hormone levels (such as hot flushes) will settle down as hormones stabilize at their new levels, when the transition is complete. But symptoms caused purely by a shortage of reproductive hormones (such as vaginal dryness) will continue.

Hormonal hiccups – the theories

Does it matter exactly what causes the ups and downs of the menopause? It does if you're planning to treat the symptoms, whether with orthodox medicine or complementary therapies. Most drugs and supplements, and even some foods, aim to have a direct effect on hormone levels. You need to be sure you're boosting the right ones.

This is something that's best tackled by a doctor or other women's health expert, backed up by your own in-depth research. Please see Chapters 8–10 on HRT, other medical help and complementary therapies before using any product.

▶ **Oestrogen deficiency** – *This was the description given to the menopause back in the 1960s, when oestrogen-only HRT was expected to keep women young into old age. The most classic sign of menopause is when you stop having periods, and this is a direct result of not producing enough oestrogen to keep the menstrual cycle going. But now that hormones are better understood, we know that it's not the only factor causing symptoms.*

▶ **Oestrogen dominance, or the progesterone theory** – *Just as menopausal problems were once blamed on a shortage of oestrogen, a later theory claimed they were caused by too much oestrogen, especially in relation to progesterone. According to the 'oestrogen dominance' theory, the body stops making enough progesterone at an early stage of perimenopause. As progesterone is the main hormone that balances oestrogen and its effects, this leaves oestrogen levels unhealthily high, especially during the two weeks leading up to a period. (Although this makes quite a lot of sense as far as it goes, it has not yet become mainstream belief. It almost certainly is still only part of the story.)*

▶ **FSH and LH** – *The 'faulty thermostat' is one of the most common and irritating effects of the menopause, causing hot flushes, night sweats and sudden changes of temperature. One theory is that, as the ageing follicles react less speedily to the stimulation of FSH and LH, the body increases its production* of these hormones to try to provoke a response. FSH and LH are controlled by the same part of the brain that regulates temperature, and high levels are believed to make the blood vessels dilate, causing a rush of heat. At the same time, the blood vessels are weakened by lack of oestrogen, which used to keep them strong and elastic, hence a sudden hot flush.

▶ **Individual sensitivity** – *This could explain why so many women's symptoms don't seem to fit the hormone status suggested by blood tests. Some women's bodies are more sensitive than others to changes in hormone levels. Some will react more to particular fluctuations or combinations.*

▶ **Xenoestrogens** – *Accidental by-products of the chemical industry, these hormone-like substances have polluted soil, water and air throughout the world. Because they're so similar to our real hormones, they can trick their way into our bodies' hormone receptors. But once there, they have very different effects. In smaller creatures such as fish, they can even cause males to change sex. In humans, they have been linked with increasing rates of cancers, especially breast cancer. Some people suspect that, as our own oestrogen production dwindles, we may be more susceptible to xenoestrogens taking its place – with all kinds of symptoms caused by their much more powerful effects.*

Insight

Xenoestrogens are hormone-disrupting chemicals found in common products such as pesticides, detergents and plastics. You may reduce your exposure, for example by avoiding plastic food containers, vinyl, PVC, harsh cleaning products and dry cleaners. Eat as organically as possible, especially meat and dairy foods.

Hormone tests

These are more likely to be carried out if you're under about 40 and there's a risk that you're going through premature menopause. High FSH levels would suggest this.

If your LH levels are high in relation to FSH, this may be a sign that you're not in premature menopause but have another condition such as polycystic ovary syndrome.

But some women's health experts recommend tests whenever you seem to be entering the perimenopause, for example, when your periods become irregular at any age. This is because your progesterone levels may be low, and high levels of unopposed oestrogen may be harmful to health.

Levels of FSH and LH normally start to increase from your early forties, and show that the perimenopause is under way.

Insight

Levels of follicle-stimulating hormone (FSH) and luteinizing hormone (LH) increase during the perimenopause, so tests can be done to see whether it's started – useful if you're planning a pregnancy. But levels of these hormones, especially FSH, can vary greatly within a day. So a single test may not be reliable.

It's like starting your periods, when you don't know what's going on

'My first experience was in a van with some other people,' says Ros. 'I suddenly thought: "Isn't it hot in here all of a sudden?" I later realized that this was my first hot flush. No one else seemed to be getting hot! It was a bit akin to starting your periods, when you don't really know what is going on and are not prepared.

'Then, some years later, I was in a car driven by my cousin, who was about 67 at the time. She suddenly said, "Open the window!" so I did. "Open it fully!" she said. She was suffering a bad hot flush at that age. She had been on HRT but was no longer. It seems the flushes may return if you take and then stop HRT – though luckily that doesn't happen to everyone. I was shocked that flushes can continue so late in life.

'I have managed to sail through the menopause, but I know people who have had night sweats and then had to teach a class of 30 kids the next day. Luck, I suppose.'

Hormones and your weight

The body produces many other hormones as well as those involved with childbearing. Some of these are also affected by the changes that happen during the menopause. One of the effects noticed by most women at this time is a tendency to gain weight, even if they had never done so before.

As you approach the menopause, changes occur in several of the hormones that control the way the body deals with food. Some of these hormones are involved in digestion; others determine whether food is used as fuel or stored as fat. And the reproductive hormones themselves play a role in increasing weight. This is partly as a result of the body's efforts to keep things functioning steadily despite the changes that are happening.

▶ *Trying to keep up oestrogen levels as the amount produced by the ovaries starts to decline, the body naturally seeks other sources. As fatty tissue produces a small amount of oestrogen, the body creates and stores as much fat as possible.*
▶ *Testosterone and growth hormone both help the body build lean tissue, which burns calories far more effectively than fat does. The more muscle you have, the more you can eat without gaining weight. Levels of both these hormones drop as the menopause proceeds.*

- *Progesterone helps the body excrete excess water. As progesterone levels start falling early in the perimenopause, many women suffer from fluid retention. This isn't actually weight gain, so it should ease off as hormone levels settle down.*
- *The thyroid undergoes temporary changes during this time too. This butterfly-shaped gland in your throat plays several roles in regulating the body's metabolism. Although a severely underactive thyroid is unusual, the gland quite often becomes a bit sluggish in women over 40. This causes symptoms that can be mistaken for those of the perimenopause, most noticeably weight gain, tiredness and confusion. In some women it becomes overactive, causing hot flushes and heart palpitations.*
- *Cortisol is a stress hormone that the body seems to produce in larger amounts during the time leading up to the menopause. It gives a quick burst of energy, but when you don't really need to run or fight, it remains in the bloodstream. As well as its discomfiting effects on mood and wellbeing, cortisol makes the body hold on to fat.*
- *Leptin is a hormone that controls the appetite and helps the body burn calories. It becomes less efficient during the menopause.*
- *Insulin regulates the amount of sugar, or glucose, in your blood. As you get older, and particularly after the menopause, the body becomes less sensitive to insulin, a condition known as insulin resistance. Instead of ushering excess glucose into the liver, insulin remains in the bloodstream where it can cause serious health problems including blood clots and hardened arteries. Insulin resistance may be more to do with age than female hormones, as this happens in men over 50 too.*

The rest

Sometimes, in trying to understand how the human body functions, we risk oversimplifying an incredibly complex organism. It's a mistake to see the body as a machine with simple parts, each playing a set role.

The body's endocrine system is immensely vast, subtle and complex. Although labelling various elements helps us to understand their roles, it also risks hiding their complexity. The hormones we call 'reproductive', for example, don't just affect the sex organs. That name covers just a few of the many functions they carry out. They are major players in so many areas that it would be pointless to try to describe all their different roles.

It helps to know this when you encounter some otherwise baffling symptom. Why does the menopause make you hungrier? One reason is that a shortage of oestrogen reduces your gall bladder's effectiveness in sending signals to your stomach that you've eaten enough. Strange but true – and the same holds for many other seemingly unrelated symptoms.

Another complicating factor is that our bodies respond differently to changing hormone levels. What triggers violent hot flushes in one woman will have no effect on another. And no one quite knows why, except that it's just a question of the individual brain's sensitivity to a hormonal change.

Having this information doesn't stop you feeling hungry, or putting on weight, or sweating with inner heat. But it can help to know it's neither 'all in your mind' nor something going wrong. You're simply coping with a force of nature.

Summary

We produce all kinds of hormones, in various amounts, throughout our lives. A few of these, the main reproductive hormones, dwindle as we reach the end of our child-bearing years. This can have a surprising number and variety of effects, because the reproductive hormones are major players that also affect many of the body's other systems. Some other hormones also change or become less efficient during this time.

The menopause isn't just about lack of oestrogen. It's the changing levels and balance of different hormones (especially of oestrogen and progesterone) that cause many symptoms. Once your hormones have settled into their new balance after the menopause, you shouldn't have any more symptoms caused by hormonal fluctuations. Any symptoms you still have will be caused by a shortage of certain hormones, especially oestrogen, and by the ageing process.

Action plan: understanding what is happening

1 *If the menopause is causing you any problem, read on to decide what sort of action to take.*
2 *You need to know your levels of different hormones if you intend to take hormone-based therapies, whether orthodox or alternative.*
3 *Blood tests are useful. However, they don't always give an accurate picture, because your hormone levels may fluctuate from one day to the next.*
4 *You may need to do some detective work. Read up on what hormonal situation is likely to be causing your particular symptoms. Consider keeping a diary to help you keep track of the changes.*

10 THINGS TO REMEMBER

1 *Hormones are chemicals that the body produces to send messages from one part to another.*

2 *Numerous different hormones are involved in all the body's functions.*

3 *The reproductive hormones – including oestrogen, progesterone and others – are those that allow a woman to conceive and carry a baby through to birth.*

4 *Oestrogen has many properties, nourishing many of the body's tissues as well as promoting fertility.*

5 *When out of balance, oestrogen can cause mood swings and irritability as well as physical symptoms.*

6 *Progesterone tends to balance the actions of oestrogen.*

7 *Many other hormones are also involved, including the 'male' hormone testosterone, which increases women's sex drive.*

8 *Menopausal symptoms (such as mood swings) are often caused by levels of different hormones fluctuating in relation to each other.*

9 *Some symptoms (such as vaginal dryness) are caused by a drop in levels of oestrogen.*

10 *Oestrogen is still produced after the menopause, although in smaller quantities than before.*

3

Physical effects

In this chapter you will learn:
- *how the menopause affects your body*
- *what else may cause the symptoms you're experiencing*
- *what, if anything, you need to do*
- *why weight gain isn't necessarily about food.*

Our bodies go through a constant process of change and adaptation throughout our lives. That's the same for both men and women. Some of these stages happen more suddenly than others. Puberty, for example, causes upheaval in most people's lives just as they're reaching their teens. After that, though, the changes happen at a less noticeable pace for men. Their hormone levels change with age too, but what's been called the 'male menopause' or 'andropause' is a gradual process. Men may remain able to father children until the day they die. Various other physical changes take place steadily in both sexes.

But because reproductive hormones have more marked effects on women's bodies – think of the menstrual cycle, pregnancy and birth – the end of a woman's child-bearing years also takes place more noticeably. The end of monthly bleeding is just the most obvious sign of the menopause. For some years before that, most women will have noticed changes in their menstrual cycles, and perhaps in other areas of their life and health.

How the menopause affects your body

The symptoms described in this chapter may look like a dismal list, but hardly anyone experiences all of them. Some are more common than others. Most women have just a few, and they rarely cause much of a problem.

However, some symptoms of the menopause may also be caused by other conditions, which may need treatment. A few of these conditions can be serious, and should be diagnosed and treated as early as possible. Some could strike at any time of life, but become more common as you get older. Some are exacerbated by the hormonal changes happening at midlife. It's important to recognize these, rather than putting everything that happens at this time down to hormones.

Don't take it for granted that anything is a natural effect of your time of life. Always go to your doctor if you have a new symptom that lasts for more than a few days.

- ▶ *To help with diagnosis, make a note of anything new you've been doing, even if it doesn't seem related to the symptom.*
- ▶ *Have you recently started (or stopped) taking a medicine or vitamins?*
- ▶ *Have you changed jobs, accepted any new responsibilities or taken up a new activity?*

The more information you can give your doctor, the clearer the route to a correct diagnosis.

Top tip

Many drugs and complementary remedies can cause side effects or interact with each other. When you're seeking a diagnosis for a new symptom, tell your doctor everything you're taking, including the dosage. And always read the patient information sheets.

Changes in the menstrual cycle

The clearest sign of the menopause is when your periods stop.
A few women find this happens quite suddenly, but most go
through a slowing down process for several years beforehand.
The gaps between periods become longer, until they finally
fade out.

Insight

Because the spaces in between periods can last several months
towards the end, it's not safe to say the process is complete
until you are sure there's not going to be another one. (You can
still become pregnant months after your last period.) That's
why the date of menopause is only known retrospectively.
A year after your final period (two years to be on the safe
side, if you're under 50), you know that you went through
the menopause a year ago.

For many women, periods become shorter and lighter as the
menopause approaches. They gradually dwindle away over a
space of a few years. This is often a sign that hormone levels are
changing quite gradually. So if this is your experience, you may
be in for an easy transition with very few symptoms.

If you're not yet in your forties when your periods become irregular,
or they stop suddenly when you're not pregnant, see your doctor.
This could be a sign of a hormonal problem such as polycystic
ovaries, which needs to be treated.

Heavy periods

Some women's periods become longer, heavier or more painful
as they approach the menopause. Heavy periods are especially
common in the early stages, when progesterone levels – which help
the womb shed its lining – are dropping. Low progesterone levels

allow the lining to go on growing for longer before it comes away, causing a heavier blood loss.

If your periods become unusually long or heavy, don't take it for granted that it's a sign of the menopause. Heavy or unusual bleeding can be a sign of several other gynaecological conditions that may need treating. You should seek a diagnosis if you often start a period less than three weeks after the previous one started, or continue for more than six days, or if you're soaking through a heavy-duty tampon or pad within a couple of hours. Losing blood between periods or when making love should also be investigated.

Heavy blood loss can be caused by growths such as fibroids, which form in the wall of the uterus itself, or polyps, which form in the cervix or the womb lining. Fibroids and polyps aren't dangerous in themselves, and some women have them for years without even knowing. But they can also be intensely painful, and may cause miscarriage if you become pregnant.

Heavy blood loss could also be caused by endometriosis, a condition in which tissue from the womb lining grows in other parts of the abdomen. Though this may spread over a large area without the woman knowing, it can also cause bleeding outside the womb along with intense pain and infertility. Less commonly, it could be a sign of certain cancers, or of endometrial hyperplasia, an excessive growth of womb-lining tissue inside the womb, which can lead on to cancer.

Whatever the cause, heavy bleeding causes a loss of important nutrients from the body, most notably iron. This is why women having heavy periods become exhausted and weak – at any time of life, let alone when dealing with other elements of the menopause.

▶ *This loss of iron can lead to anaemia, which can be serious and needs medical treatment, usually in the form of iron supplements.*

▶ *Get your doctor to do a blood test to check this really is the
problem, rather than just taking iron tablets, which can cause
other problems such as constipation.*

▶ *Iron stores can also be replenished by eating foods that are
rich in either iron itself or the other nutrients that help the
body use iron most effectively. See Chapter 12 on nutrition
for more information.*

Premenstrual syndrome (PMS)

PMS can be difficult to pin down, as there are so many possible
symptoms. The emotional effects are well known: mood swings,
irritability and fits of depression. But the physical effects include
headaches, nausea, fluid retention, breast pain and swelling –
and these could have numerous other causes. As with any new
symptom, don't try to diagnose it yourself: go to your doctor.

During their thirties and early forties, some women develop PMS
for the first time, or after being free of it for many years. Others
suffer many of the same symptoms as part of the hormonal
changes leading up to menopause. Does it matter which is the
case? Yes, for several reasons. If you're planning to become
pregnant in the future, you need to know whether you've started
the perimenopause, as your fertility will be declining steeply.
Or if you're starting an early menopause, taking action in good
time could prevent harmful effects.

▶ *One way of working out if your symptoms are more likely to
be PMS or perimenopause is to check the timing. Keeping a
diary may help with this.*

▶ *The symptoms of PMS usually begin during the last few days
before a period starts, although bad cases can begin up to two
weeks before. The symptoms usually stop as soon as a period
starts, often quite abruptly.*

▶ *When the same symptoms are caused by the menopause,
they can stop and start at any time throughout the menstrual
cycle.*

I felt scarlet, though I only looked pink

'My major worry was the hot flush,' says Val, who is now retired. 'I always became very self-conscious because I felt I was glowing like a fire engine – I was certainly generating enough heat! I was an actress in those days and got very panicky at the thought of having a hot flush during a job interview, or while I was on stage or some other really public occasion.

'One day I felt a flush coming on and fled to the ladies' loo to hide. In the big mirrors I was suddenly aware that although I felt as if I looked scarlet, in fact I only looked a little pink. I found that very comforting. Thereafter, I always ignored the flushed feeling and waited for it to pass. By seeming to be relaxed I stopped attracting attention to myself and managed to get through it.'

Vasomotor symptoms, or the faulty thermostat

The 'vasomotor symptoms' are the most notorious signs of the menopause: hot flushes ('hot flashes' in the USA) and their nocturnal equivalent, night sweats. They seem to be caused by a sudden drop in oestrogen levels. It doesn't necessarily mean oestrogen levels are low at this time – the drop could be from very high to moderate levels.

For some women this is an early symptom, when oestrogen levels are generally still high, suggesting that it's caused more by the sudden change than by lack of oestrogen in total. At this stage, you're most likely to have a hot flush in the last week before your period starts, which is the time when oestrogen levels are low. However, they are most common around the time when periods stop altogether, and for a year or so afterwards. As the perimenopause progresses and your oestrogen levels decline, hot flushes may happen at any time of the cycle.

No one is quite sure why a drop in oestrogen has this effect. One theory about hot flushes is that fluctuating hormone levels make the brain more sensitive to tiny increases in temperature. Blood vessels at the skin's surface then dilate in a rush to release what your body thinks is dangerously excessive heat. It's certainly true that keeping cool can prevent hot flushes in many cases.

But whatever the reason, you experience a sudden rush of heat, particularly in the face. It's real and measurable; your temperature actually does go up a couple of points, and a severe hot flush can leave you drenched in sweat. That's what has happened when you wake up covered in perspiration at night. You may even feel dizzy or faint because of the sudden temperature change. Severe hot flushes can disrupt your life.

This faulty menopausal thermostat is the most common reason for using HRT. In the worst cases, debilitating hot flushes can make it hard to hold down a job.

But your way of life plays an important role too. You're twice as likely to suffer from vasomotor symptoms if you smoke. Being overweight or suffering from anxiety also increase the risk. Alcohol, hot drinks and spicy food can trigger a hot flush. Because of this, many women find vasomotor symptoms respond to the kind of do-it-yourself measures found in Chapters 10–13 on complementary approaches, lifestyle, nutrition and fitness. Anything that relieves stress, for example, is going to reduce the number and severity of hot flushes.

▶ *Hot flushes may be caused by a few other conditions such as an overactive thyroid or certain cancers. As always, go to your doctor if you have any suspicions.*

- Hot flushes can also be caused by chemotherapy for breast cancer, or certain drugs for depression, anxiety or high blood pressure. In this case, your doctor may be able to tailor the dosage to reduce side effects.
- Ironically, hot flushes can also be caused by selective oestrogen reuptake modulator drugs, or SERMs, such as raloxifene. This is prescribed to reduce the risk of osteoporosis – making it an alternative to HRT.

Sleep deprivation was the hardest experience

'It started when I was 48 years old. At night I would lose precious sleep, tossing and turning and being drenched in perspiration,' says Margaret, an artist who retrained as a life coach in her fifties. 'During the day I experienced the typical sweating and red face, with my temperature seeming to change rapidly from my feet right through to the top of my head. But sleep deprivation was the hardest experience, as I was working 12-hour days.

'My weekends were spent trying to catch up on much-needed rest, but the cycle of night sweats prevented me from enjoying more than two hours' solid sleep at any one time. The sleep pattern is now so fixed that, even though I am well and truly through the symptoms of menopause, I still wake every two hours. Thank goodness there's no sweating!'

Central nervous system

If you find yourself dropping plates, losing balance and tripping over your feet, it may come as a relief to find out that you're suffering from nothing more serious than the menopause. It's surprising, till you stop and think that hormones regulate all kinds of physical functions, including those associated with the central nervous system.

Because some of the other possible causes could be serious, do tell your doctor what's worrying you and ask for tests. These will probably rule out conditions such as multiple sclerosis or Parkinson's. But if they don't, you have a much better chance of keeping these under control with an early diagnosis. Other possibilities are ear problems, including tinnitus (noises in the ear), which often starts at about this age. Clumsiness or loss of balance can also be caused by stress, low blood sugar from skipping meals, or just being in too much of a hurry.

Once you've ascertained that your new-found clumsiness really is just caused by your time of life, it's surprisingly easy to alleviate. Exercises such as t'ai chi and yoga improve your balance and coordination. If you'd like individual advice, you may find a physiotherapist who will work on a tailored set of exercises with you.

This is also the time of life when some women suffer from 'restless legs', an irritating condition in which your legs start twitching and jumping for no apparent reason. Men can also develop this condition, although it is less common. Some people get an unpleasant sensation building up before the twitching occurs. It's worst at night, and may stop you sleeping.

Restless legs can be caused by iron deficiency, or the brain's inability to use iron, so get your doctor to check your iron levels – don't take supplements unless you're certain you need them, as it's dangerous to have too much iron in your system. It may also be linked with diabetes or kidney disease. There are drugs for this condition, but they all carry side effects. Like so many other midlife symptoms, it's safer, and often more effective, to treat restless legs with lifestyle changes.

Other effects of hormonal changes on the brain and nervous system include a string of psychological disturbances (see Chapter 4 on mind and mood), insomnia and heart palpitations.

It hardly needs saying that you should report changes in your heart rhythm to your doctor. Women tend to feel safe from coronary heart disease before the menopause, because it's seen as a men's disease. But it can strike young women – even non-smokers – and the risk increases sharply after the menopause. In fact, more women die of heart disease than of any other condition.

Almost all the physical conditions stemming from hormonal effects on the brain and nervous system can be relieved. Turn to Chapters 11–13 on lifestyle, nutrition and fitness for suggestions on how to do it.

Breast symptoms

Many women notice pain, swelling and/or lumpiness in their breasts at various times, most often in the week or so before a period starts. These symptoms become more common during the hormonal changes of the perimenopause. The good news is that, like other long-standing hormone-related conditions, these symptoms may actually stop once you've passed the menopause.

Insight

Among these common conditions are breast fibroids, or fibrocystic breast changes. These feel like little separate lumps that move under the fingers, giving rise to their informal name of 'breast mice'. Although they're not cancerous in themselves, they may increase your risk of breast cancer. It's not a large extra risk, but knowing about it could actually protect you, by reminding you to stay in tune with your body and take notice of any changes.

Breast pain and swelling are also quite common as hormones fluctuate. This sort of pain affects both breasts equally, with a feeling of bloated tenderness. It isn't a sharp pain and doesn't affect the nipples. It tends to happen regularly, usually just before a period – though as the menstrual cycle becomes irregular, the symptoms may also crop up at unexpected times.

These symptoms are usually nothing more serious than hormonal changes. All of them may respond well to lifestyle and nutritional changes, and some complementary therapies. Sometimes a change of contraceptive pill helps. Starting HRT may make these symptoms worse, in which case you should try other formulations.

Breast symptoms that are not normal include discharge, or a new pain or a change in appearance or feel, especially on just one breast. (See Chapter 11 on lifestyle for details.) Any of these symptoms could mean serious conditions, including infections and cancer. Go to your doctor for a diagnosis, as prompt treatment can cure them. Although minor breast pain isn't usually a sign of cancer, don't put up with it if it changes or becomes persistent. And if you develop breast tenderness after you start taking HRT, this can be an early warning of cancer.

It's good to become familiar with the normal shape and feel of your breasts, so that any change is quickly picked up. If you do notice a change, don't waste time wondering – go for a check-up. It's unlikely to be breast cancer, but it really isn't worth taking the risk.

Digestive and urogenital symptoms

Pregnancy often causes constipation, and some women have loose bowel movements during a period. In the same way, the hormonal changes of the perimenopause can affect the digestive and eliminatory systems.

Be wary though, as a change in bowel habit can be an early sign of diseases including colorectal (bowel) or ovarian cancer.

So if you have constipation or diarrhoea, or notice a change in the look or feel of bowel movements, report this to your doctor. Although bowel cancer is common, it can be cured if diagnosed early enough. You're more at risk if a close family member has had it; if you've had chronic constipation or ulcerative bowel disease; or if you smoke or consume a lot of alcohol or meat.

Constipation is quite common at this time of life. But once you've had cancer ruled out, constipation should be easily relieved by lifestyle changes, including diet and exercise.

Indigestion, too, affects many women, especially later in the perimenopause. But it's a bit harder to deal with. Various hormonal changes affect your appetite and sense of satiety. The gall bladder becomes less efficient, and as one of its functions is to send the stomach a signal that you're full up, you simply go on feeling hungry. At the same time, the stomach may be emptying more slowly, which means it's easy to overload it. In addition, hormonal changes weaken the muscle that acts as a valve at the top of your stomach, preventing acid from leaking up towards your mouth. That's why acid reflux and heartburn are common problems at this time. See Chapter 12 on nutrition for how to deal with these symptoms.

One of the most unwelcome effects of the menopause, for many women, is urinary incontinence or urgency. Again, it's because hormonal changes weaken the muscles that hold everything in place inside. This comes as a shock, especially to women who haven't had children and thought it would not affect them. Some women find they leak urine when they laugh or sneeze. Others have so little warning of needing to urinate that they can't get to the bathroom in time. It can be so distressing that women become reluctant to go outdoors, or wear large pads every day.

But there's no need to live with urinary incontinence. Special exercises can tone up the muscle that's given way, and these days there are numerous products that also help. If all else fails, a small operation can cure the problem. See Chapter 7 on sexuality for more information.

Dryness

Oestrogen has a lubricating effect, helping to keep skin and membranes in good shape. As oestrogen levels fall, around the time when periods stop, many women experience a drying-out effect. Skin and hair lose their shine. Some women get what seems to be eczema, but is simply caused by drought conditions.

Even eyes can become dry, causing tiredness and soreness; some women can no longer wear their usual contact lenses. Dry eye syndrome, which can affect both sexes, is most common in women over 40.

This dryness can also lead to urogenital problems, such as thrush and urinary infections. Vaginal dryness causes difficulty with love-making. In the bladder, the irritation it causes can exacerbate urinary incontinence or urgency.

HRT can delay some of these effects, although as they're caused by a shortage of oestrogen they will return when you stop taking it. If you would like to prevent the vaginal dryness without signing up for the whole HRT experience, you can try hormone-replacing creams or pessaries. Similarly, lifestyle changes and simple remedies can help with the other drying effects.

Perhaps surprisingly, HRT doesn't necessarily help with dry eyes. In fact, women who are taking HRT (especially oestrogen alone) suffer more from dry eye syndrome than those who aren't.

Pain

Pain is another of the unexpected symptoms of the menopause. Headaches and migraines, breast pain, achy joints and muscles are fairly common at this time. Any of these symptoms could be a sign of other conditions, so, as usual, new symptoms should be reported to your doctor and not ignored. One of oestrogen's many benefits is believed to be reducing inflammation. So when oestrogen's protection disappears, your body suddenly notices the results of long-term wear and tear.

Insight

In recent years, the cholesterol-lowering drugs called statins have become so popular that they can now be bought over the counter. It is becoming recognized that statins often cause muscle pain, so if you're taking statins and become aware of constant or frequent niggling muscle pain, don't automatically blame your hormones. Ask your doctor for a creatine kinase (cK) blood test. High levels of this enzyme are caused by muscle damage – stopping the statins may help to put them back to normal.

Fatigue

A lot of women feel tired and run-down during the menopause. It's not surprising, given everything that can be going on at the same time. Heavy periods and other hormone-related problems are just one element. Women in their forties and fifties are often working, looking after a houseful of teenagers, caring for elderly relatives – sometimes all at the same time.

But constant tiredness can also be a warning sign of numerous health conditions, some related to the menopause and others not. Some of them are serious and need treatment. Don't take it for granted that you'll feel fine again once you've got through this busy time – you may well do so, but in the meantime why suffer?

Heavy periods, for example, cause a debilitating loss of iron from the blood. But taking supplements (especially minerals, such as iron) often makes matters worse by causing imbalances. If you take iron tablets and hope for the best, you could be masking important warning signs of a more serious condition. And if the iron tablets give you a bit of extra energy for a while, they may delay a life-saving visit to your doctor.

Insomnia is a frequent problem at this time of life, sometimes caused or made worse by menopausal night sweats. But how do you know this is what's making you so tired? Exhaustion is also one sign of heart disease or an underactive thyroid. Would you know the difference?

If cutting down your workload or getting to bed earlier has no effect, seek a diagnosis. Find out what is causing your tiredness – even if it's nothing serious, your doctor should be able to come up with something more specific than 'it's just your time of life'. If it's not serious enough to need medical treatment, try the relevant chapters in this book for further advice. As exhaustion makes the mental and emotional symptoms of menopause worse, Chapter 4 on mind and mood offers suggestions for dealing with it.

Insomnia responds well to lifestyle changes. Chapters 12 and 13 on nutrition and fitness also offer many options for improving your energy levels.

Weight gain

It's hard to avoid putting on a bit of weight during the menopause. This is the result of many different hormonal changes. Some hormonal changes increase your appetite, some reduce your ability to burn off calories and some increase the body's tendency to store fat. For a fuller explanation of why it happens, see Chapter 2 on hormones, and for what to do about it, see Chapters 11–13 on lifestyle, nutrition and fitness.

Putting on weight around the middle is a common result of low oestrogen levels. By the time your periods have stopped, weight tends to gather around your midriff instead of in the classic younger woman's 'pear shape', on hips and thighs. This new 'apple shape' – common among men as well as among women after the menopause – is associated with an increased risk of heart disease and diabetes. It's not just an outward sign of internal changes, either. That midriff fat is itself harmful to your heart, unlike fat on other parts of the body. It is chemically active, playing a role in increasing potentially harmful fats such as cholesterol and triglycerides.

If you can't shake off all those extra kilos, though, there's one consolation: fat cells produce a weak form of oestrogen. So carrying just a little extra weight could be counteracting some of the ageing effects of the menopause.

Sometimes what looks like weight gain on the abdomen, especially in the early stages of perimenopause, is actually fluid retention. A shortage of progesterone makes the body store fluid in the tissues. This causes a puffy swelling that's less solid than fat and may also show up on other parts of the body such as the arms and face. If low progesterone levels are the cause, the swelling may fluctuate during the menstrual cycle and should wear off by itself as the menopause continues and your body adapts. But don't take this for granted. Fluid retention – especially around the wrists and ankles – can also be a sign that the heart isn't functioning effectively.

Insight

If a white mark remains for a moment after you press a finger into your flesh, you probably are retaining fluid. It should ease off by itself after periods stop.

A thickening of the waist can also be a sign of osteoporosis – though this is much less likely. This condition makes bones (including vertebrae) become brittle and break more easily. The damaged spine then becomes compacted and the back therefore looks shorter and wider. Luckily, osteoporosis is quite unusual until well after the menopause, except in women with specific risk factors such as eating disorders. Excessive dieting can disrupt hormone levels to the extent that periods stop; if this has ever happened to you, your bones have been subject to the same conditions caused by the menopause. So if you notice that your waist looks thicker even without a general weight gain, ask your doctor for a bone scan.

Changes in the thyroid gland's efficiency can also make you put on weight. It sometimes becomes slightly underactive during the menopause. This slows down your metabolism, making you pile on weight while feeling slow and lethargic. A serious thyroid malfunction, which is much less common, would cause a particular pattern of weight gain – moon-shaped face, puffy eyes, possibly a swollen neck – along with other symptoms such as thinning hair, hoarseness and feeling cold.

Top tip

If you're troubled by symptoms that come and go, keep a diary to help you work out what triggers them. Include everything you eat, your activities and the time of your menstrual cycle.

Summary

The hormonal changes of the menopause can cause numerous symptoms. The list of possible effects looks daunting, but most women only experience a few, and not severely. Many of the symptoms could also be signs of other health conditions, though. And if you're taking medicines, a 'symptom' could actually be caused by a side effect or interaction. So don't presume that any new symptom is a harmless, temporary effect of the menopause – go to your doctor for a diagnosis. Once you've ruled out other, more serious causes, use the later chapters of this book to find options that will help you.

Action plan: know what you're dealing with

1 *If you're having what you suspect is a symptom of the menopause, check in this book to see if that's likely.*
2 *Have any new symptom checked by your doctor – especially if it causes pain.*
3 *Turn to later chapters to find out how to treat any inconvenient symptoms, both medically and with self-help measures.*
4 *If you are still having periods and need to lose some weight, make an extra effort to do so now. It's much more difficult to lose weight after your periods have stopped.*

10 THINGS TO REMEMBER

1 *Most women only get a few menopausal symptoms, if any.*

2 *Hot flushes are the best-known symptom of menopause, but there are many others.*

3 *Periods usually become irregular, but may not become lighter – some women have heavier periods in the early stages of perimenopause.*

4 *Some symptoms may be unexpected, such as joint pains, insomnia or loss of balance.*

5 *The digestive system is strongly affected by hormonal changes at this time, as is the ability to control weight gain.*

6 *You may need to try several different treatments or self-help options to find what works for you.*

7 *There are effective treatments for all menopausal symptoms, including the long-term ones.*

8 *The most effective and long-lasting solutions are usually the self-help options.*

9 *Don't presume any new symptom is a sign of the menopause, as some health changes at this time may be unrelated.*

10 *Several diseases become more common at this time. Breast and bowel changes, in particular, may be perimenopausal or may be a sign of cancer.*

4

Mind and mood

In this chapter you will learn:
- *how hormonal changes temporarily affect your outlook*
- *what other factors may affect your mind and mood at this time*
- *safe and effective ways of dealing with emotional disturbances.*

The perimenopause can be a difficult time in a woman's life. And it's not 'all in your mind' – hormones affect the whole of your body, including your brain. You may even start to wonder if you're suffering from mental illness, although this is unlikely. The mind and mood symptoms you may encounter at this time are likely to have one of the following causes:

- ▶ *hormonal effects on the mind and emotions, such as mood swings, despondency and possibly even memory lapses*
- ▶ *your natural response to circumstances – being upset when things go wrong isn't an illness!*
- ▶ *lifestyle factors such as exhaustion, stress and nutritional deficiencies*
- ▶ *other health conditions, where the symptoms may be similar to those of the menopause*
- ▶ *depression – it's less likely than the other causes, but can strike during the perimenopause.*

There are many ways of coping with these effects. To start with, it helps to know what's causing your particular experience. If you are encountering difficulties at this time, read on to see how best to deal with them. This chapter includes specific advice for dealing with the non-physical symptoms of the menopause. In addition, Chapters 8–12 on remedies and self-help consider non-physical as well as physical symptoms.

Most encouraging of all, scientific studies have shown that, for women, the risk of depression peaks in the forties and then falls – often lower than in their youth. After your periods stop, and for the rest of your life, you are less likely to suffer from depression than before you started the perimenopause.

Hormonal effects on emotions

Emotional problems can be a reaction to common prejudices about this time of life. One prejudice is about women being ruled by their hormones. A widespread misunderstanding of menopause means that it's seen by many people as a major disruption, equivalent to a nervous breakdown. Women are almost expected to become irrational, moody and depressed. And when that's expected, and you're feeling tired or bleeding heavily, it's easy to oblige.

It is true, however, that hormones can directly affect your emotions. What happens is probably that progesterone and oestrogen affect the brain's production of neurotransmitters – chemicals that (among other functions) influence emotion.

MOOD SWINGS

Rapidly fluctuating hormone levels can cause abrupt changes in your mood, similar to those that some women with PMS experience just before a period. These sudden mood swings can have a disorienting effect.

You can find yourself too angry to speak one moment, then close to tears the next. You are fully aware of how irrational you're being, but the feelings are frighteningly out of control. Very few women actually become violent, but many have to bottle up a simmering rage. It feels horrible and can wreck relationships at work, with friends, with a partner, even with your own children – especially if they're going through their own teenage hormonal battlefield.

LOW SPIRITS

Hormonal fluctuations shouldn't last too long. But there is also a steady decline in hormone production as the perimenopause continues. Because hormones such as oestrogen have effects on the brain that make you feel happier and more energetic, lower levels can lead to sadness and lethargy. You no longer enjoy what used to be your favourite activities.

But as with other aspects of the menopause, it's not just about low levels – it's also about your body's individual sensitivity and how long it takes to adapt. Your feelings should gradually lift as the body adjusts to its new balance. In the meantime, the techniques in this chapter should help you feel your best whatever the cause of your low spirits.

Some women find that HRT helps them feel better emotionally, although there's no scientific evidence of this and others say it makes them feel worse. In particular, some women find HRT causes mood swings and exhaustion as a result of renewed heavy bleeding. If you wish to try HRT but are put off by side effects, it's worth experimenting with different formulations.

'My feelings about menopause and being in my fifties are mixed with a certain sort of sadness,' says Christine. 'There is no longer the possibility of having children of my own. There is also a sense of mortality that was not there before. It tangles with a deep love of life, living and beauty, and, now, a store of memories that will die with me.'

Am I losing my mind?

One of the most unexpected and unwelcome symptoms of the perimenopause is what some women have described as 'brain fog'. You can't think clearly. You may find your concentration span shrinking too. Women's famous ability to multi-task goes out of the window. And along with these goes your ability to make and carry out decisions.

Memory is particularly hard hit, as you struggle to remember names and phone numbers. You forget what you were going to say; names vanish from the tip of your tongue. Then one day you pause at the top of the stairs and utter those dreaded words: 'Now, what did I come up here for?' At that point, many women fear they're experiencing the first signs of dementia.

Don't panic – dementia is very unlikely. Hormonal fluctuations may affect the brain, as your body's natural oestrogen plays a role in learning, memory and decision-making. Its effects on the brain include strengthening communication between nerve cells and aiding the production of neurotransmitters involved in memory.

Tiredness, stress and overwork add to the pressure for many women at this time. All of these pressures can leave you feeling your brain is losing its grip.

Insight

To some extent the brain symptoms are temporary. They are partly to do with circumstances, physical symptoms and your body's sensitivity to hormonal changes, which will settle down after the menopause.

The good news is that you can sharpen up your brain by exercising it – and this will go on working after the menopause to help counteract the ageing process. Like any other form of exercise, the more you work at it the better the results. You can do this with any kind of mental stimulation, from crosswords or card games to Open University courses or career retraining. You need to vary the activities, or you could just become a demon card-player who still can't find her keys.

The brain effects of menopause may be frightening now but once your postmenopausal balance is established, you may even look back and laugh. Meanwhile, take some practical measures to make your life easier.

HOW TO GET YOUR BRAIN BACK IN GEAR

The cloudiness should wear off by itself eventually. Meanwhile, you need to cope with temporary difficulties in concentrating and remembering. Also, keep your brain active to stop things getting any worse. Many books and websites offer helpful advice. Here are some of the most immediately useful tips:

▶ *For important tasks, write a to-do list and keep it somewhere visible. Cross tasks out as you go along, and make a new list each week so it never becomes illegible.*
▶ *Some websites give valuable advice and support in getting organized. Why not bookmark one that you like and visit it regularly?*

- *If you haven't used a diary before, keep one now. A week-per-view format – the sort that shows you seven days on two facing pages – helps you organize each day in the context of the whole week. If you need more space, use a taller book or one with a page per day, rather than making notes too small to read. For the household, buy the kind of large calendar that has separate space for each family member, keep it near the front door and tell everyone it's their responsibility to keep their own section updated – and to look at it. Use just one diary and one calendar.*
- *Keep a computer file or a page in your diary for each activity or organization you're involved with. Add new names and other important pieces of information before you can forget them.*
- *Give up multi-tasking. From now on, put your mind to whatever you are doing and complete it before starting another task. If you feel you have too many things to do, are you sure you couldn't line them up and take them one at a time? When that's really not possible, give your main attention to anything that could be dangerous if you make a mistake.*
- *For all everyday tasks that you have to get right, set up routines for yourself. Get into the habit of, for example, always hanging your keys on a hook in the kitchen when you come in, and always stopping on the way out to check you've picked them up. You can adapt the details to suit your own way of life – keep a set of keys in every handbag, or hang them anywhere that a burglar can't reach with a wire through the letterbox. The important thing is to do the same thing every time.*
- *For other activities, take the opposite approach in order to give your brain some exercise. Do something different every day: take another route to the shops, buy your lunch from a different deli, try a new exercise class. This actually builds new pathways in your brain, exercising it as effectively as you can exercise muscles.*
- *Try to put a few moments each day aside to organize. Finding more effective ways to manage your time can give you an extra hour or more in each day. But don't burden yourself with impossible aspirations.*

- *Try taking up meditation – see Chapter 10 on complementary approaches. It's been shown to improve focus and concentration at any age. Also, by relieving stress, it prevents anxiety from building up and making you feel even more confused.*
- *Some women find that HRT helps. You shouldn't go on taking it for years, but it could buy you time to start feeling the benefits of making some healthy lifestyle changes. On the other hand, some studies, including the large-scale Women's Health Initiative (more about this in Chapter 8), suggest that taking HRT may actually increase the risk of dementia. These researchers were looking at women who were taking HRT when they were over 60, so we don't know how it would affect younger women.*

Insight

Hormonal changes can have confusing effects on the brain and emotions. But of all menopausal symptoms, these are among the most amenable to do-it-yourself solutions. Slotting some simple self-help techniques into your everyday routine can make a noticeable difference within a very short time.

Your natural response to circumstances

Many women feel sad, anxious or resentful at this time. And why not? This is a time of transition that you may not welcome. No one over the age of 20 wants to be reminded that they're getting older. But natural though these feelings are, they don't help you get through any difficulties you're encountering.

GRIEVING

If you're feeling sad at this time, there's also a realistic element of mourning. Every life change involves the loss of what you had before. That may be easy to give up when you've chosen to make the change, but it's hard when change is forced on you.

No matter how reluctant you would be to have a child in your fifties, for example, the end of fertility is a loss like any other. It's natural to experience some sadness or mixed feelings. Women who have children may feel this loss as keenly as those who haven't.

Loss of youthful status is also painful. Images of youth and beauty are everywhere, making an older person seem not just less valuable but almost abnormal. While this affects both sexes to some extent, and decades of feminism have improved women's options, men still have many more escape routes than women, through higher-status occupations and more acceptance of older male faces. Menopause is an inescapable reminder of our increasing age.

Being perfectly honest, most people feel some pangs of regret as they reach this time of life. You have every right to accept your feelings and briefly mourn the passing of time. But it doesn't have to be a big deal. Eternal youth would have been nice, but this is what we've got and we'll make the best of it. There's even a hidden bonus. If you've slipped into a rut, this is a good moment to take stock. You're still young enough to set new goals, or achieve those you put aside when career or children took up all your energy.

FAMILY CONCERNS

Many women going through the menopause have elderly parents who may be losing their health and independence. This is not only a practical concern but a potential source of great anxiety, and a painful recognition of their frailty. Children are growing up and moving away. Women may also be dealing with changes in their own or their partner's health, long before they were expecting this to be a problem.

The menopause comes at a time when long-standing relationships may be tested by one partner's efforts to recapture lost youth. The breakdown of a long-term relationship at any age causes massive grief and upheaval. This is all the more true when you're going through hormonal changes that can make you feel old and unloveable. It can cause as much pain as bereavement. Sometimes it feels as if you are faced with many kinds of loss.

On the other hand, you may have a houseful of teenagers going through their own hormonal upheavals. You try to be patient, but really it's not the easiest time in your own life. Or your grown children may still be living with you, at a time when you had hoped to have some more space. Don't feel bad about wanting to meet your own needs as well as everyone else's.

WORKPLACE PRESSURES

All this comes at a time when increased competition in the workplace is putting pressure on women as well as men. If you've been earning your own living for the past 20 to 30 years, it comes as a jolt to realize how dispensible you are to your employers. You may not define yourself purely by your occupation, but are you happy to be sidelined in favour of keen young rivals? If you haven't yet received the promotion or other recognition you hoped for, it may not be going to happen.

There are practical solutions to some of these issues. At work, for example: if your job is causing stress and unhappiness, look at your options. If career is not a top priority, work out your finances very carefully and ask yourself if you still need to be putting so much into a job. Could you afford to go part-time? If it is a top priority, look into extra training or refreshing your work skills to stay on top. Also, ask yourself how much satisfaction you're getting in comparison with the stress. This isn't a good time to walk out on a job, if you want to go on working, but there's nothing to stop you looking for a new one while you're still employed.

Remember that you also have a right to mourn what you're losing. You don't have to pretend none of it bothers you. The workplace isn't a good spot for getting things off your chest, as this is likely to make matters worse. Find the right surroundings to talk through your feelings and grieve if you need to. This could be with close friends, especially if they're going through similar trials. Various forms of counselling can be very helpful at this time. Online forums offer a chance to talk things through with people in the same situation. However, if you're talking through intimate matters

with strangers online, do be very careful to maintain anonymity –
both your own and that of your workplace and people you mention.

Lifestyle factors

Sometimes, the pressures of everyday life add to the challenges
posed by hormonal fluctuations. It can be difficult to keep up a
healthy way of living at the best of times: find out more about how
to do it in Chapter 11 on lifestyle. Pressures that tend to make the
mind and mood symptoms worse include stress, exhaustion and
nutritional deficiencies.

STRESS

Everyone knows stress is bad for you. It has particularly negative
effects on your emotions when you're already coping with
hormonal changes.

Stress also affects the cognitive functions of your brain. Have you
noticed how you make bad decisions when you're under pressure?
It's not just because you're having to do things in a hurry and
getting muddled. The stress hormones, such as adrenaline and
cortisol, have powerful effects on your brain. This is exactly what
they're meant to do when you need to make a sudden escape from
danger. But like anything that's meant for use in emergencies only,
they're harmful when used too often.

Chronic stress can damage your brain. You'll start to notice you
can't think clearly any more, and you're less effective at carrying
out tasks or remembering what to do. If you feel trapped, and
powerless to change whatever is causing all this stress, it can also
lead to serious depression.

Some of the advice in this chapter should help you reduce the
amount of stress in your life. See also Chapter 10 on complementary
approaches for advice on meditation and other ways of relaxing.

EXHAUSTION

The perimenopause starts at a busy time in most women's lives – when they are still caring for children, often concerned with elderly relatives, earning a living and running a household. It's a lot to hold together. A work or family crisis and a few nights of insomnia may be all it takes to cause overload. Menopausal crises are often triggered by exhaustion.

Insight

Hormonal changes affect women's sleep patterns in several ways, reducing the ability to drop off or to stay asleep, or triggering disruptive night sweats. The resulting tiredness exacerbates many symptoms of the menopause, especially those of the brain (such as difficulty concentrating) and emotions.

The first and simplest solution to exhaustion is to get more sleep. Adults need at least seven hours' sleep a night until they reach old age. If you're under any kind of stress, you'll benefit from more.

Another part of the solution is to try to reduce your workload. Can sisters or brothers help care for your parents? Do you really need to drive your children everywhere now that they're old enough to use public transport? (Travelling with others of their age helps children build up social and practical skills.) If you can't get other family members to help with housework, could you live with some dust building up, or afford to hire a cleaner?

If, on the other hand, you feel tired no matter how much you sleep, you should go to your doctor. Constant unexplained tiredness is an early symptom of many diseases – and an early diagnosis gives the best possible chance of successful treatment. If you're lethargic despite sleeping long hours, you may be suffering from depression.

Read Chapter 11 on lifestyle to find out how to get a good night's sleep.

NUTRITIONAL DEFICIENCIES

Your need for certain nutrients increases when your body is under pressure from hormonal fluctuations. A shortage of necessary nutrients can affect your mind and mood as well as create physical symptoms.

You may overlook this issue on the grounds that you're eating a healthy diet. But if you're not getting enough of the particular foods you need during this stage of life, you could be feeling the effects. Even if not serious enough to cause harm by themselves, nutritional deficiencies can exacerbate an existing problem. See Chapter 12 on nutrition for more information.

ALCOHOL

Alcohol isn't unhealthy in itself. In fact, a lot of research shows that drinking in moderation is good for your health and may increase your life expectancy. A glass of wine with dinner or a couple of drinks while you're out with friends are among life's harmless pleasures. But beware if you find you need a drink to help you unwind after a hard day. It's all too easy to slip into drinking too much when you're under stress.

Mood swings and problems with concentration are warning signs that you're drinking more than your body can cope with. If you're getting memory lapses too, you need to bring your drinking under control.

Once confident, I started to question myself

'At the beginning of menopause I experienced a vulnerability unlike any other,' says Margaret, now in her late fifties. 'I often questioned my basic knowledge, skills and decision-making, especially at work. This, for a once-confident

woman, I found very disconcerting! The feelings of
vulnerability gradually passed and my confidence eventually
returned.'

Margaret was an accomplished dancer who practised
several times a week. 'I really believe that my exercise
routine at the time, plus a very positive outlook on life,
got me through the depressing times. Daily exercise
not only meant that my bones were strong, but it also
cured depression, anxiety and stress. I believe a positive
attitude to life is essential in maintaining good health,
both physical and mental.'

Other health conditions

As with physical symptoms, effects on your mind and mood could
stem from other causes. Symptoms of some diseases could be
mistaken for those of the perimenopause.

Alzheimer's is the first thing most of us think of when we can't
remember a relative's name, or if we're unable to decide whether to
have tea or coffee. In reality, any kind of dementia is uncommon,
especially before the age of about 60. Forgetfulness and difficulty
in making decisions are more likely to be caused by tiredness or
stress, though they can also be a sign of depression.

Some drugs can also affect the brain, especially those such as
tranquillizers that aim to alter your mood. If you have become
forgetful or confused since you started taking a medicine, it's
important to tell your doctor.

Mood swings can have a few non-hormonal causes, including
undiagnosed sleep apnoea (a condition that causes unrefreshing
sleep) and certain brain conditions. Otherwise, they are most likely

to be just your body's individual reaction to the normal hormonal changes of perimenopause.

Watch out for two health conditions in particular, which become more common at this time of life. A number of mind and mood symptoms, including forgetfulness and mood swings, may be an early sign of either diabetes or thyroid dysfunction. Both of these can be controlled more effectively if picked up at an early stage, so it is worth asking your doctor to do tests.

Top tip

The herbal remedy St John's Wort works as an antidepressant for mild to moderate depression. However, it does have some side effects, and it can interact with other drugs including antidepressants and contraceptives. See Chapter 10 on complementary approaches for details, and consult your doctor if you are already taking any medicines.

Depression

In rare cases, things get worse than just feeling down. If you've been unhappy for months, are lacking in energy (without any physical reason) and are feeling life isn't worth living, you may have sunk into a state of real depression. One of the tell-tale signs is an inability to enjoy anything, even your favourite activities or relationships.

In addition, depression includes at least four of the following symptoms:

- ▶ *feelings of guilt or worthlessness*
- ▶ *memory lapses and inability to concentrate*
- ▶ *loss of energy*
- ▶ *thoughts of suicide or death*
- ▶ *either agitation or slowness of movement*
- ▶ *sudden change in appetite or weight*
- ▶ *insomnia or excessive sleeping.*

Although depression usually wears off by itself, it may take weeks or months. In the worst cases, depression may need medical treatment.

In some cases, known as dysthymia, the condition continues for years like a chronic, low-grade infection. Dysthymia is defined as a depressed mood for most of the day, occurring most days, and lasting at least two years, again without any underlying physical illness. It also includes at least two of the following symptoms:

- *loss of appetite or overeating*
- *insomnia or excessive sleeping*
- *low energy or fatigue*
- *low self-esteem*
- *difficulty concentrating or making decisions*
- *feelings of hopelessness.*

If you feel trapped in depression or dysthymia, you may want to consult your GP. Many people have been helped by psychotherapy or counselling. Antidepressants have helped some people through a particularly bad patch of depression. However, these drugs should not be a first resort, as their side effects can be harmful (including an increase in the risk of stroke among women after menopause) and you may become dependent on them quickly. See Chapter 9 on other medical help for more information.

Insight

It's a myth that women suffer more from depression after the menopause. It is most common in earlier life. However, women sometimes encounter it as a temporary symptom, often along with mood swings, during the perimenopause.

DON'T HURT YOURSELF

If you feel suicidal at any time, you should seek help at once. Go to your doctor and say exactly how you're feeling. If things are so desperate, antidepressant drugs may help you through, although some people feel worse for the first few days. Go to your doctor or hospital at once if you feel worse. Be very careful not to come off antidepressants suddenly, as this has been known to trigger a sudden suicidal crisis.

Helplines that offer non-judgemental counselling or listening include:

- *The Samaritans, UK 08457 90 90 90, Ireland 1850 60 90 90, www.samaritans.org, jo@samaritans.org*
- *Australia: Lifeline, 131114*
- *USA: 1-800-SUICIDE*
- *Contacts and helpline phone numbers in 40 countries: www.befrienders.org*
- *Online forum: www.walkers.org.*

Top tip

If depression has dulled your appetite, or if you're eating junk food for comfort, make a commitment to nurture yourself. Healthy eating not only gives you energy but can also relieve low spirits or mood swings.

BEATING THE BLUES

The most effective way of relieving sadness or long-term dysthymia is to find ways of bringing happiness, or at least contentment, back into your life. Much of the advice doctors give, about getting out and taking exercise, is aimed at breaking the cycle of unhappiness. It's when people feel too lethargic to do so that they return for antidepressants. Unless you feel suicidal (in which case, please seek help at once), do try some of the well-researched techniques below before taking antidepressants.

Scientists have done some wonderfully simple and effective research into happiness. Instead of focusing on theories, they have asked people what actually made them happy. This research has been carried out by teams of scientists all over the world, and the results are very similar.

One essential piece of advice is to decide you want to be happy and make a commitment to achieve that goal. It may sound simple and obvious, but few people actually do it. Set aside some time every day to work on your goal of happiness, even if it's as little as a ten-minute break spent eating your lunchtime sandwich in the garden.

This is a serious project, and you may need to do some work. Keep notes of what you find is working, or of obstacles if you encounter any. Make an effort to organize each of the activities below. Jot down how you feel after you do each one, just to see which activity is having the best effects.

▶ *Take notice of what you're doing when you feel happy. Identify the activities that make you happy and spend more time on them. Don't wait for things to happen – take the initiative and organize them.*

▶ *Take your mind off your problems. If your thoughts keep returning to your depressing situation, find something to distract yourself. Gnawing over and over the same problems doesn't lead to a solution. If there's something you can change, you have a better chance of discovering it if you come back to the subject refreshed. Meditation can help, as long as you keep ignoring all intrusive thoughts.*

▶ *Spend time with upbeat people that you like. The more you enjoy your social life, the less possible it is to suffer from depression. Don't waste time with those who bring you down, or make you feel burdened, or see the cloud behind every silver lining. And don't rely on other people getting in touch – set up meetings yourself.*

▶ *Share your troubles, but only briefly. Getting things off your chest can help a lot, as can helping a friend through hers. But resist the urge to wallow in your grievances.*

▶ *Have fun. Laughter triggers the release of pain-killing, mood-lifting hormones that make you feel better instantly. Even anticipating laughter reduces your body's production of stress hormones. It just has to be what scientists call 'mirthful laughter' – nothing subtle or satirical.*

▶ *Be active. Taking part in any lively exercise, whether it's an aerobics class or kicking a ball with the kids, increases your body's production of feel-good endorphins.*

Summary

The menopause can have disturbing effects on your brain and emotions. Problems at this time may have a hormonal basis, or they may stem from physical symptoms of the menopause, or from other conditions. Low moods may also be a realistic response to changes in your life. And exhaustion is common at this age, when you're busier than ever but with less energy to spare. If you're unhappy, try breaking the cycle with some of the well-researched self-help techniques now available. If you're seriously depressed, your doctor should be able to help – and you must definitely seek help if you feel suicidal. This chapter offers advice for coping with mind and mood symptoms, whatever the cause. Follow these tips to be happier, more effective and clearer in your mind.

Action plan: smoothing out any temporary blips

1 *If you're experiencing any mind or mood problems, try to identify the cause.*
2 *Unless you need to see a doctor for a diagnosis, try the self-help measures in this chapter and later in the book.*
3 *Make a commitment to yourself to build up your happiness and keep your brain in good shape.*
4 *If things don't improve within a couple of months, or if they get suddenly worse, seek medical help.*

10 THINGS TO REMEMBER

1 *The hormonal upheaval of perimenopause can cause a number of emotional effects such as mood swings.*

2 *These are often compounded, during your forties and fifties, by numerous work and family concerns.*

3 *The emotional effects should settle down by themselves after menopause – though there's no need to wait, as there are many ways of counteracting them.*

4 *Decide on your emotional goal (for example, to be happy) and make a commitment to doing something towards it every day.*

5 *Hormones can also have disruptive effects on the brain, including forgetfulness and an inability to concentrate.*

6 *Because the brain effects are unexpected, they can be frightening. Don't worry – it's very unlikely to be dementia.*

7 *Although the 'brain fog' should ease off after menopause, it's better to tackle it as you go along so that it doesn't become entrenched.*

8 *Getting organized is the first step towards bringing brain fog under control.*

9 *Some women find that hormone replacement therapy (HRT) helps with the brain symptoms, although this hasn't been backed by published evidence.*

10 *Antidepressants are major drugs with potentially dangerous effects. St John's Wort is more likely to ease mild depression, with less drastic side effects.*

5

Midlife health

In this chapter you will learn:
- *what conditions become more of a risk at this time*
- *how to calculate your individual risk*
- *how to take action to avoid them.*

The perimenopause provides women with a unique health opportunity. Men can easily drift through middle age without noticing any changes, until they're suddenly felled by a heart attack. For women, midlife changes happen suddenly and unmistakeably. This abrupt change may be unwelcome at the time, but it can actually save lives.

Our changing hormone levels affect numerous bodily processes, some of which are unconnected with reproduction. As a result, this is a time when we may get warning signs of health conditions that could become serious if unchecked. These early warnings allow us to take action in good time – creating even better health than we had before.

Conditions to look out for at this time include:

- ▶ *some cancers*
- ▶ *diabetes*
- ▶ *coronary heart disease*
- ▶ *thyroid disease*
- ▶ *osteoarthritis*
- ▶ *osteoporosis.*

Most of these conditions are exacerbated by the hormonal changes around the menopause. Fortunately, you can strongly reduce your risk of any of these conditions by taking action now. It's really worth making the few lifestyle changes that could prevent these common problems bedevilling your later years.

If you have any of the risk factors listed in each section below, you may want to let your doctor know and ask for advice. They're not all equally significant, and in most cases your doctor is more likely to recommend healthy lifestyle changes than medicines. But don't take this for granted: tests may reveal something that can and should be treated at an early stage.

Top tip

Be aware of any unexpected changes in your body or your health. You don't need to do set self-checks, just know your own body and be sensitive to any differences.

Breast cancer

It's the disease women tend to fear more than any other, and most of us know the statistic that one in eight women will develop breast cancer. As with a lot of other cancers, your risk of developing a breast tumour increases as you get older.

However, breast cancer is not the biggest killer: heart disease, for example, kills many times more women. And the menopause, which reduces your body's production of oestrogen, slows down the growth of cancers that are fuelled by oestrogen. This includes certain kinds of breast cancer, along with some cancers of the reproductive system: ovary, endometrium and cervix.

Much of your breast-cancer risk is determined by forces outside your control, such as family history or the number of periods you've had (fewer is better, in this case). But not all breast cancers are genetically linked, and those that are tend to strike at an earlier age. A healthy lifestyle can reduce your risk of developing breast cancer from other causes. The risk reduction may not be as dramatic as the way stopping smoking slashes your risk of lung cancer and heart disease, but it is especially protective as you get older.

HRT increases the risk of breast cancer, though experts are divided about how much the risk is increased. If you're in a high-risk group, you may prefer to err on the side of caution and avoid taking HRT. But if you want to take HRT, it's something you should discuss with your doctor. Read more about this in Chapter 8 on HRT.

You may have an increased risk of breast cancer if:

- ▶ *your mother, sister, aunt or grandmother had cancer of the breast or ovary*
- ▶ *you have benign breast disease (such as fibrocystic breast changes – non-cancerous lumps)*
- ▶ *you had a first pregnancy after the age of 30*
- ▶ *you have never breastfed a baby*
- ▶ *you drink more than two units of alcohol a day*
- ▶ *you reached puberty early, had a late menopause or have never been pregnant*
- ▶ *you take HRT.*

Insight

Your chance of developing midlife conditions depends on many factors including your lifestyle, your medical history and any diseases that run in your family. You can get some clues by asking, for example, what your grandparents died of and, if a blood-relative has had cancer, what type it was.

WHAT TO DO

You can reduce your risk of breast cancer significantly by staying a healthy weight, not drinking too much alcohol, cutting down on saturated fats and taking some exercise on most days.

Keep an eye on any changes in your breasts, by doing a quick check when you undress or are in the bath. Look out for any changes, especially a lump or puckering of the nipple. Your partner can help too, by letting you know if they notice any changes.

Go for regular mammograms – from 50 onwards in the UK, you should be invited for one every three years – and ask your doctor about the results. Lumps can be removed with very little damage to the surrounding area, and early treatment for breast cancer is increasingly successful.

Cancer awareness

Breast cancer isn't the only cancer to be aware of. Without becoming obsessive, you can keep an eye open for early signs of the common ones. Never presume that fatigue, bloating or back pain is just a sign of menopause; never accept that a change in bowel habit is just irritable bowel syndrome (IBS) without tests being done.

Have your cervical smear test every three years until the age of 50, and every five years after that. Keep track of it yourself rather than relying on your GP to call you in.

Ask for an anaemia test every year or so, especially if there is bowel cancer in your family. Anaemia can be a sign of internal bleeding.

Be aware of any moles on your body, especially your legs (where women most often develop melanoma; men get it more often on their backs). Notice any growth or irregularity or other changes, and report them to your doctor. Removing a mole is quick and easy, and a biopsy will be done to see whether it was cancerous.

Diabetes

There are two main kinds of diabetes: type 1, which used to be known as juvenile or insulin-dependent diabetes, and type 2, formerly known as adult-onset diabetes. The names have changed largely because type 2 is becoming widespread among children too.

The incidence of diabetes is increasing, in all age groups, as our average weight increases. Women's risk of diabetes rises sharply after the menopause. But it is even more strongly linked with excess weight, especially when it expands your waist size into an unhealthy 'apple shape'.

Our bodies turn food into glucose, or sugar, to use as fuel, as well as producing some in the liver. Normally, the amount of glucose in the bloodstream is regulated by a hormone called insulin. What happens in diabetes is that the body either can't produce enough insulin to control blood-sugar levels, or becomes unable to use it effectively. Excessive amounts of glucose can injure the internal organs, cause nerve damage and lead to death if not treated. Fortunately, diabetes can be controlled with injections of insulin, drugs or a special diet.

The classic sign of diabetes is frequently visiting the loo, as your body tries desperately to offload the excessive glucose through urine. This in turn makes you constantly thirsty. Fatigue, unexplained weight loss, hunger, blurred vision, skin disorders and odd feelings in your fingers or toes are other symptoms. But be wary: you can develop diabetes without noticing any symptoms at first.

You may have an increased risk of diabetes if:

- *you are overweight, especially around the middle – this is the biggest risk factor for women at this age*
- *any of your close relatives have diabetes*
- *you have had blood-sugar problems during pregnancy*
- *you have given birth to a baby weighing more than 9 lbs*

- *you have had polycystic ovary syndrome*
- *you have high cholesterol or triglyceride levels*
- *you have high blood pressure (more than 140 over 90)*
- *you lead a sedentary life*
- *you are of African or Asian descent.*

WHAT TO DO

If you have any hint of problems with your blood-sugar levels, see your doctor at once. In fact, if you're overweight or have other high risk factors, it may be worth getting a blood test anyway. Blood tests will quickly show whether you have diabetes, or are slipping towards it.

The good news is that you have a very good chance of preventing diabetes, even if your blood-sugar levels are already high. For most people, the most effective route is to lose weight and increase daily activity. Research has found that these lifestyle changes work much more effectively than drugs.

Even if you have developed diabetes, healthy eating and exercise may help you control it without drugs. But don't try to go it alone. Diabetes can be life threatening, so do follow medical advice. Your doctor will probably be delighted to help you tailor a healthy lifestyle programme.

Insight

Of all serious conditions that become more common at midlife, it's probably easiest to make a substantial reduction in your risk of diabetes because it's very much linked with unhealthy diet, excess weight and lack of exercise.

Heart disease

During the past few years, doctors have discovered that heart disease often affects women differently from men, and as a result women's symptoms are frequently mistaken for those of other conditions, or not noticed at all. Medics have only recently started separate research on women with heart disease, so a lot of information has yet to start filtering through.

When people speak about heart disease in middle age or later, they usually mean the most common kind: coronary heart disease, or coronary artery disease (sometimes abbreviated to CHD or CAD). It happens when the coronary arteries – the vessels that supply blood to the heart – become blocked, usually with a build-up of plaque on the walls. Despite its image as an old person's disease, it often strikes in middle age.

Women tend to feel safe from this as long as they are having periods. And it's true that coronary heart disease becomes a lot more common among women after the menopause. But it's a myth that you can't suffer from it before your periods stop. Many women have been startled by a diagnosis – or worse, a heart attack – before they've had any signs of perimenopause.

In women, the signs of heart disease often include insomnia, fatigue, mild breathlessness or pains that can be taken for heartburn or indigestion. Because these could be caused by other conditions, they don't ring immediate alarm bells. Although the sharp chest pain called angina is a classic sign of heart disease, many women with the disease never experience this and others feel a sharp or dull pain in the shoulders, back or even the jaw instead.

Even a heart attack may not give women the classic crushing chest pain, breathlessness or pain down the arm that most people would recognize. Though either sex can have any of the signs, a woman is more likely than a man to feel a pain between the shoulder blades, indigestion or nausea, recurring chest discomfort or a sudden weakness. And don't discount your inner wisdom: women who survive heart attacks often say they felt an inexplicable sense of dread before any physical symptoms.

You need to be aware of these signs as you get older, because heart disease is so common that being in a low-risk group doesn't mean you won't develop it. Smoking is one of the major risk factors, but non-smokers aren't immune, even before the menopause. Similarly, although high blood pressure is a warning sign, plenty of people with heart disease have normal blood pressure. The role played by stress is increasingly recognized – but heart disease can also strike the most relaxed people.

Women do tend to put on weight round the middle after menopause. Doctors are now concerned about what is sometimes called the metabolic syndrome: a large waist measurement; abnormal triglycerides and low HDL (the 'good' cholesterol); high blood sugar; and high blood pressure. People who have this collection of symptoms have a high risk of going on to develop heart disease.

You may have an increased risk of heart disease if:

- ▶ *coronary heart disease or high cholesterol runs in your family, especially in women*
- ▶ *any of your relatives (especially women) have been diagnosed with heart disease before the age of 60*
- ▶ *you have high blood pressure*
- ▶ *you have diabetes*
- ▶ *you had an early menopause, whether this was natural or caused by chemotherapy or removal of your ovaries*
- ▶ *you smoke*
- ▶ *you have ever been severely underweight, for example through anorexia*
- ▶ *you suffer a lot from stress, anxiety or depression.*

WHAT TO DO

Have your blood pressure, cholesterol and blood sugar checked every year. But don't worry too much if your cholesterol is slightly above the preferred 5 mmol/litre. Women tend to have more of the good cholesterol (HDL) than men, so overall cholesterol measurement is less important.

Smoking and stress cause the most risk. So giving up smoking and dealing with stress are the best lifestyle changes you can make for

your heart. The bonus is that this will improve your health in many
other areas too.

> ## Top tip
> If you suspect you're having a heart attack, dial 999 and then
> chew an aspirin with some water. The aspirin thins the blood
> and can dissolve a blockage, and chewing gets it into your
> bloodstream faster.

Thyroid disease

Are you feeling the cold more than usual, or finding it hard to
summon up any energy? Thyroid problems are more common
in women than men, and often start around the time of the
menopause. The most common kind is underactivity, or
hypothyroidism, although overactivity and other conditions can
also occur.

The thyroid, a butterfly-shaped gland in the throat, produces
hormones that help control the body's metabolism. It's not
uncommon for production to slow down in women over 40. This
can cause symptoms that are easily mistaken for those of the
perimenopause. These include constant fatigue, weight gain, low
moods, muscle pain or cramps, constipation, dry skin, depression
and indecision.

About a third of women taking HRT find it doesn't help their
symptoms. Endocrinologists have suggested that, in some cases,
this is because the symptoms are either caused or made worse by
an underactive thyroid.

If you suspect this is happening, you can get a friend to help you
check your neck for changes to the thyroid. You tip your head back
and swallow a mouthful of water. Your friend should be looking at
your throat just below the adam's apple, to see if any protrusions
become noticeable as the water goes down. (You can do this for

yourself by looking in a handheld mirror, but you could still use a friend to bang you on the back if you choke.)

The most visible sign of a serious thyroid deficiency is a goitre, or swelling in the throat. It's often caused by lack of iodine in the diet, or occasionally by an excess of iodine. It's rare except in some undeveloped inland areas where iodine doesn't occur naturally and isn't added to salt. In a developed country, hypothyroidism is more likely to be caused by an autoimmune inflammation of the gland.

This is not the only sign of thyroid trouble, though, and many women have an underactive thyroid without any swelling in the throat.

You may have an increased risk of thyroid disease if:

▶ *you have had thyroid trouble in the past*
▶ *you have a family history, especially in your mother or sister*
▶ *you have had any autoimmune disease*
▶ *you have taken iodine supplements or had any medical treatment including iodine (other than simply swabbing some on a wound)*
▶ *you smoke or have smoked in the past*
▶ *you are on a salt-free diet.*

WHAT TO DO

If you are concerned that your 'menopausal' symptoms are caused by an underactive thyroid, ask your GP for a blood test to check levels of thyroid-stimulating hormone. If yours are low, you may be prescribed replacement hormones. But if after a few months your symptoms haven't significantly improved, do ask your doctor whether you need to keep taking the medicine.

Certain foods, described as 'goitrogenic', contain compounds that increase the risk of a goitre in people who are already at risk, especially if you eat them raw or in large amounts. These include cabbage, Brussels sprouts, broccoli, radishes, cauliflower and kale.

If you're at risk, consider cutting them out of your diet. But don't cut them out unnecessarily, as this family of foods is otherwise one of the healthiest you can eat.

Some people are concerned that soy may affect the functioning of the thyroid. There isn't a lot of evidence to suggest that it does, but if you're in a high-risk group it might be best to avoid eating a lot of soy products, especially those in concentrated form such as supplements. Unless your doctor tells you differently, though, it should be safe to eat normal soy foods such as miso or tofu. See Chapter 12 on nutrition for details of the debate about soy.

Arthritis

There are many forms of arthritis, but by far the most common is osteoarthritis. It's what causes the pain that many women start to notice in their joints – most especially their knees – during their forties. Osteoarthritis is so common that it's usually known simply as 'arthritis'. (Rheumatoid arthritis is an autoimmune disease, very different from osteoarthritis and much less common.)

Researchers have found that osteoarthritis can be triggered by changes in oestrogen levels. They don't know exactly why this happens, though, or why it affects women's knees more than their other joints. What we do know is how to reduce the risk and damage.

Although arthritis is usually described as being caused by 'wear and tear' – or use and injuries – researchers have found that the 'tear' element is far more important. Just getting older is much less of a hazard. Weight-bearing exercise, such as walking or even running, shouldn't cause any harm as long as you don't overdo it.

It's the injuries, large and small, that cause arthritis. And the perimenopause is a time when hormonal effects on the central nervous system make many women a little accident-prone.

Arthritis causes pain, stiffness and/or swelling in the joints. Though not life threatening, it can be severely painful and restrictive. Pain in the joints when the weather is damp is an early warning sign.

You may have an increased risk of osteoarthritis if:

- ▶ *you have ever had an injury, especially of a joint*
- ▶ *you are overweight*
- ▶ *you regularly carry out heavy work or repetitive movements*
- ▶ *you lead a very sedentary life*
- ▶ *older members of your family have arthritis.*

WHAT TO DO

It is important to try to avoid accidents that could hurt a joint, such as tripping and landing on your knees. Don't become cautious in your movements, though, as this reduces your activity at a time when it's important to stay active. A better solution is to take exercise that strengthens your muscles and improves your balance: see Chapter 13 on fitness.

Along with injuries, the other main risk factor for arthritis is being overweight. So this is a good time to lose any extra kilos before they start pressing on your joints.

If you have been diagnosed with arthritis, your doctor may prescribe painkillers. Try not to take these every day, as they not only become less effective but you can also become dependent on them and lose your body's natural ability to cope with pain. A study by researchers at Queen Mary University of London in 2008 showed that pain-relieving creams are just as effective as tablets but with fewer side effects.

The Arthritis Research Council (and many GPs) recommend supplements that have been found to ease arthritic pain: 1500 mg a day of glucosamine sulphate or 1500 mg a day of cod liver oil.

A large trial is currently studying the effects of 400 mg a day of vitamin D supplements on arthritis.

Osteoporosis

Much has been written about osteoporosis during the past few years. Most of us now know that women's bones become thinner and more brittle after the menopause, increasing the risk of a fracture. Hip joints can snap and vertebrae suffer a series of small fractures, each unnoticed at the time it happens.

We're often urged to remember the little old ladies we saw as children, whose backs were bent like a question mark – a sad sight that we're not likely to forget. But remember that those little old ladies were born in hard times, living through wars and depressions. They are much more likely than anyone reaching middle age now to have gone hungry and missed the chance to build up strong bones.

Osteoporosis mainly affects elderly people, especially if they're very thin or not eating well. Among younger people it usually stems from eating disorders or over-exercising. In midlife, you can keep your risk down by walking every day, taking weight-bearing exercise, eating healthily, including calcium-rich foods such as dairy products, and not getting too thin.

How much of a problem is osteoporosis for most of us? The terms 'osteopenia' and 'pre-osteoporosis' have come into use, suggesting that having bones that are below optimum density is a health condition in itself. But as the standard of bone density is measured in young women, most women past the menopause will fall short. However, this doesn't mean they're likely to suffer a fracture within the next couple of decades.

Also, new research is suggesting that it's not just about bone strength or density. Bone-mineral density hasn't been found to predict who is most likely to suffer a fracture. Many women who suffer fractures have quite good bone density; their bones become less resilient for other reasons, which are still being explored.

Falling down is an important risk factor for broken bones in older people, according to a paper published in the *British Medical Journal (BMJ)* in 2008. The best way to prevent this cause of fractures in later life is to build strength and balance, ensure you're getting enough calcium and vitamin D and avoid drugs that cause dizziness.

That's not to say that osteoporosis isn't a concern. It does become a problem with increasing age, and it can strike younger women whose bones have been weakened by crash-dieting or other risk factors. If you actually have osteoporosis, it can be treated with drugs.

But major medical organizations such as the British Medical Association are warning that much concern about osteoporosis is being created by the drug manufacturers. A report in the *BMJ* warns that 'although public promotion of those drugs often relies on presentations of relative reductions in fracture risk, the absolute reductions for healthy women are small when weighed against potential harms and costs.'

HRT also gives the bones some protection, if you start it early and keep taking it for at least five years. But its usefulness is limited. Doctors usually recommend stopping HRT within five years because it increases the risk of other serious conditions including breast cancer. It's a question of weighing up what you're most at risk of.

Also, your osteoporosis risk increases to normal when you stop taking HRT. Most fractures happen to women over 75 – long after we are advised to stop taking replacement hormones. So HRT is exerting its protective effects during a relatively low-risk period, not when you most need them.

You may have an increased risk of osteoporosis if:

▶ *your mother had a hip fracture before the age of 75*
▶ *you're Asian – black women have the lowest risk, white women are in the middle*
▶ *you're small-boned or underweight, or have often crash-dieted*
▶ *you smoke*
▶ *you ever stopped having periods, except during pregnancy or the perimenopause*
▶ *you had an early menopause*
▶ *you lead a very sedentary life*
▶ *you use certain medicines every day, such as steroids (say for asthma), SSRI antidepressants or thyroid drugs (diuretics and indigestion remedies containing aluminium may also steal the calcium you need to keep your bones strong)*
▶ *you have certain conditions such as diabetes, rheumatoid arthritis, chronic inflammatory bowel disease, hyperthyroidism or coeliac disease.*

WHAT TO DO

By far the best way to prevent osteoporosis is to keep your bones strong through healthy eating and weight-bearing exercise. Supplement this with strength and balance training to prevent falls (see Chapter 13 on fitness).

Calcium is important to keep bones strong, and is plentiful in dairy produce. Vitamin D is also essential, and is created by the action of sunshine on your skin, so take as much of that weight-bearing exercise outdoors as possible. In temperate climates such as northern Europe, avoiding the midday summer sun should be enough to protect you from skin cancer. Your doctor may prescribe calcium and vitamin D supplements if necessary.

If in doubt about your osteoporosis risk, your GP may refer you for a Dual X-ray Absorptiometry (DEXA) scan, which measures calcium, or an ultrasound, which measures your bone density.

If you have osteoporosis or your doctor thinks you're at high risk, you may be offered HRT. Other drugs that may help are biophosphonates such as alendronate, etidronate or risedronate. These drugs have helped women who actually have osteoporosis, although their numerous and often serious side effects (such as inflammation of the oesophagus) put many people off.

Selective estrogen/oestrogen receptor modulators (SERMs) such as raloxifene (Evista) are an alternative. Raloxifene has proved moderately helpful, reducing the number of spinal fractures from ten per cent to between six and seven per cent among women taking it for three years, though it didn't prevent any other fractures. Its side effects are generally less serious than those of biphosphonates, but it can cause hot flushes.

However, these drugs haven't proved their worth as a preventive measure. And if you're taking biphosphonates, you need to ensure you're getting enough calcium and vitamin D too: the drug may even harm bone if you're short of these nutrients.

Summary

The hormonal changes around the menopause can trigger certain health conditions associated with midlife. It's possible to work out whether you are at high or low risk of developing any of them. This doesn't mean you definitely will, as many other factors (including chance) are involved in becoming ill. However, assessing your risk factor gives you an opportunity to take preventive self-help measures to reduce your risk, if you wish to do to. If you recognize that you may be suffering the first signs of these conditions, you should consult your doctor for a diagnosis. You can then make any lifestyle changes your doctor recommends, and have the condition treated if necessary.

Insight

There are drugs available that are meant to prevent certain conditions, for people considered to be at high risk. If you are offered these, weigh up the possible benefits against the risks of taking new drugs. They may not work as expected and could have unknown long-term effects.

Action plan: improving your health prospects

1 *Find out your family health history by asking older relatives about any conditions that may run in the family. Older people may not wish to speak about their own health, but should be able to tell you about relatives, especially if anyone died before old age.*

2 *Make notes of your own medical history and see if it puts you at particular risk of anything.*

3 *On the basis of what you've found out, consider taking medical advice and making lifestyle changes, if necessary, to improve your health prospects. Chapters 11–13 on lifestyle, nutrition and fitness give more details.*

4   *If your doctor thinks you are at high risk, even without symptoms, you may be offered preventive treatment. If you're not suffering and the drugs have side effects, though, think hard before taking drugs to prevent a disease you might not get anyway.*

5   *Check that you're on your doctor's list to have all the health checks you're entitled to. Ask to have tests if they are not offered.*

10 THINGS TO REMEMBER

1   Not all changes during the forties and fifties are connected with the menopause.

2   Various health conditions become more common at this time, including diabetes, thyroid disease, heart disease and some cancers.

3   You can work out your risk of some conditions from your own and your family background.

4   Remember that this doesn't tell you that you definitely will, or won't, get a disease – just whether the likelihood is high or low. Other factors also play a part, including chance.

5   With your personal risk in mind, ask if your doctor would recommend any course of action.

6   Without getting obsessive, be aware of bodily changes.

7   See a doctor about any new symptoms that you notice.

8   Have all recommended tests and check-ups carried out regularly.

9   Take self-help action where possible, for example any form of exercise that's particularly helpful in preventing a condition that concerns you.

10 Making some lifestyle changes at this time can have an enormous impact on your health and wellbeing for the rest of your life.

6

Contraception and fertility

In this chapter you will learn:
- *why your contraceptive needs change during this time*
- *how to choose a method that suits your current lifestyle*
- *what to do in case of contraceptive failure*
- *how to improve your chances of pregnancy if you want to have a baby.*

One of the mistakes women sometimes make about the perimenopause is to believe that a woman is no longer fertile when she is not having regular periods. It's true that this makes you less fertile, but you still need to use contraception if you don't want a pregnancy at this time of life. The number of births to women in their forties more than doubled from 1988 to 2010 in Britain, along with a sharp increase in the number of abortions among the over-forties.

From your late thirties onwards, your contraceptive needs may change. Your fertility starts to decline around this time, but you can get pregnant at any age as long as you're still ovulating. Even in your mid-fifties, if you're still having periods there's about a four per cent chance of pregnancy a year if you don't use contraception.

On the other hand, if you do want a baby, conception becomes more difficult once you reach the early stages of the perimenopause. Your hormones could be changing significantly before you start to notice the obvious signs such as irregular periods or hot flushes. So you should be aware of changes that mean time is running out.

When periods become infrequent, you can't be certain you're not going to have another ovulation. That's why doctors advise continuing to use contraception until one year after the last period if you're over 50, or two years after if you're less than 50. You could become pregnant by chance after your last-ever period.

Contraceptive options in the perimenopause

Hormonal forms of contraception such as the Pill are popular because they're easy to use and nearly 100 per cent effective. But they do carry the risk of some adverse effects. The worst of these is a blood clot, thrombosis, or venous thromboembolism. And like any drug, the Pill may have side effects, so you may have to try a few formulations before you find one that suits you.

Some women stay on the combined Pill throughout their reproductive life. But many have to make a change after the age of 35, if their health and other risk factors make it unwise to keep taking oestrogen. And a lot of women prefer to use non-medical alternatives, especially if they've been taking pills for over 20 years.

COMBINED ORAL CONTRACEPTIVE (COC)

This popular form of contraception is more than 99 per cent effective. It can be helpful if you suffer from painful or heavy periods. Side effects include breakthrough bleeding, breast tenderness, acne and mood swings.

The most serious adverse effect that's likely to happen while you're using the COC is the development of a blood clot. The combined Pill increases your risk of suffering this dangerous condition by up to five times. The greatest risk comes during your first year on the Pill, but it still exists later, especially if you are overweight.

You shouldn't take the Pill if you have high blood pressure, as it increases your risk of a heart attack – which becomes a concern as women approach the menopause. It also slightly increases your risk of having a stroke. Smoking while you're on the Pill increases your risk of a heart attack by up to ten times.

Staying on the combined Pill for more than five years increases your risk of cervical cancer, which is why it's important not to miss your regular cervical smear test. It also slightly increases your risk of breast cancer. However, long-term use of hormonal contraception actually reduces your risk of several cancers – of the ovary, endometrium and bowel.

Once you're past the age of 35, the health risks start increasing, so you may be advised to change your contraceptive method. Your doctor will encourage you to stop taking the combined Pill if you have migraines, or if you smoke or are obese, as these factors add to the risk.

▶ *The combined Pill suits many women throughout their forties, but should not be continued past 35 if you have oestrogen-related risk factors.*
▶ *If you want to stay on the combined Pill, this could be a motivation to give up smoking or lose extra weight.*
▶ *The oestrogen in a combined Pill works like HRT, preventing the menopausal symptoms of hot flushes, night sweats and vaginal dryness.*
▶ *Many doctors now recommend coming off the combined Pill at 50 even if you have no other risk factors. It gives a higher dose of oestrogen than HRT does. You will still need to use contraception until you find out if you have stopped ovulating.*

Insight

The oestrogen component of the combined oral contraceptive (COC) Pill works like HRT, providing steady doses of hormones. It could prevent the symptoms caused by hormonal

(Contd)

fluctuations, especially hot flushes. If you get on well with the Pill, and aren't in a high-risk group, you can stay on it through your forties.

CONTRACEPTIVE PATCH

The contraceptive patch Evra delivers the same kind of formula as in the combined Pill. It has the same benefits, side effects and risk factors. It may also cause skin reactions and headaches. One patch is left on for a week at a time; after three weeks/patches, you leave them off for a week.

> ▶ *The contraceptive patch may suit someone who dislikes swallowing tablets and has no reason to stop taking oestrogen.*

PROGESTOGEN-ONLY PILL (POP)

If you smoke or are overweight, you're likely to be recommended to swap to the POP when you pass the age of 35. The risks of taking the large doses of oestrogen in the combined Pill become much greater from then on. The POP contains no oestrogen and even less progestogen than the combined Pill. Still 99 per cent effective, the POP is only slightly less convenient.

Its low dose means you need to take it at the same time each day. If you are even three hours late, you may be advised to take emergency contraception as a back-up. Even if you haven't had sexual intercourse for a few days (as conception can take place some time after intercourse), keep taking the pills and use barrier contraception too for the rest of the month.

A newer POP, called Cerazette, containing a form of progestogen called desogestrel, may help, as it can be taken up to 12 hours late. It also suits women who don't want to have periods, as about half of all users stop having them.

Unlike the combined Pill, the POP doesn't cause blood clots. But it has the same range of common side effects as the combined Pill, with the addition that it frequently causes irregular periods and breakthrough bleeding. It also increases the risk of ovarian cysts.

When changing to a POP, start taking the new pills the day after you finish the last packet of combined Pills, without a pill-free interval.

▶ *The POP is useful for women who like being on the Pill but need to give up the oestrogen component.*
▶ *If brain fog makes you forget to take the Pill at the right time, this method is not for you.*
▶ *This method can be used to prevent periods if you wish to.*

INJECTABLES AND IMPLANTS

Progestogen-only contraception is available as injections and implants as well as pills. Convenient and highly effective though they are, their side effects make them unpopular.

Medroxyprogesterone acetate (Depo-Provera) lasts for three months after an injection. It has a lot of side effects, including weight gain, menstrual irregularity and possibly also depression. Long-term use of injectable contraception may increase your risk of osteoporosis. Another injection, norethisterone oenanthate (Noristerat) is only licensed for short-term use in the UK.

The matchstick-sized implant etonogestrel (Implanon) has to be inserted and removed by a specialist. It can be left in for up to three years, but can cause weight gain, headaches and acne.

▶ *Injectables and implants offer little benefit to anyone who can manage other forms of contraception.*
▶ *These contraceptive methods are unsuitable for any woman approaching the perimenopause who may still want to have a baby, as fertility may not return for up to a year after stopping the injections or having the implant removed.*

INTRAUTERINE DEVICE (IUD)

Another useful option is an IUD, a T-shaped plastic and copper device that sits inside the womb. It works both by releasing copper, which causes a build-up of white blood cells in the cervix to kill the sperm, and by stopping the egg implanting.

More than 98 per cent effective, it needs to be fitted by a trained nurse or doctor. But after that, if it suits you, it's even simpler than taking the Pill. It just needs to be checked after the first month, and then once a year, and it can stay in for up to ten years.

An IUD raises none of the long-term health concerns of hormonal contraception. Any ill effects are clear and immediate. There's a slight risk of infection being caused when it's inserted. If you develop a temperature, discharge or pain in your lower abdomen within the first three weeks after the IUD is fitted, go to your doctor at once. This could be pelvic inflammatory disease, which can lead to infertility and internal scarring. Even if it isn't infected, the device will need to be adjusted. And in rare cases an IUD can come adrift and need to be removed under anaesthetic.

An IUD can cause heavier periods with more discomfort. Unlike barrier methods, it doesn't offer any protection from sexually transmitted diseases. In fact, there's always a slight chance of infection entering via the threads that extend through the cervix into the vagina. Because your risk of infection increases with the number of partners you have, an IUD is safest when you're in a steady relationship.

- *If you have an IUD inserted when you're over 40, you can keep it in until you no longer need contraception.*
- *Highly reliable and convenient, this method could suit you if you're in a steady relationship and don't want to take hormones.*
- *An IUD is probably unsuitable if you suffer from period pains or heavy bleeding, as it often exacerbates these conditions. However, an IUD can be removed whenever you choose if you decide to give it a try anyway.*
- *An IUD is unsuitable if you have numerous partners due to the risk of infection.*

INTRAUTERINE SYSTEM (IUS)

This is an IUD containing a progestogen called levonorgestrel, known as the Mirena. It has proved more than 99 per cent effective as a contraceptive, and has the valuable extra effect of controlling heavy bleeding, making it ideal for women who like everything about the IUD except the heavy periods.

Like the ordinary IUD, the IUS keeps life simple. It's also suitable for women who don't want to take oestrogen. Its lifespan is a little shorter at five years.

Because it is a form of hormonal contraception, it does carry some health risks and is not suitable for women who have had cancer of the breast, womb or ovaries. It may cause side effects of abdominal pain, backache, acne, headaches and breast tenderness during the first few months. And like the IUD, there's the risk of infection.

- *The IUS may suit women suffering from heavy bleeding, although it may take some time for the good effects to outweigh the initial, temporary side effects.*
- *This method is not for anyone who dislikes hormonal contraception.*
- *If fitted after you reach 45, an IUS can be kept in until you no longer need contraception.*
- *Having an IUS allows you to take oestrogen-only HRT without risking endometrial cancer.*

An IUS changed my life

'I had heavy periods that got worse and worse for years. It was like turning on a tap,' says Sue, a 49-year-old married nurse. 'Investigations found that I had fibroids, which were probably causing the heavy bleeding. A friend had a Mirena IUS fitted and recommended it.

'It's changed my life,' says Sue. 'I can't tell you how good it is. It was for contraception, but it works just as much for heavy bleeding. You have to persevere with it; I got a lot of back pain and stomach ache at first. But once it's settled in it's an absolute dream. The doctor said the fibroids might be in the way, might prevent progestogen being absorbed. But I said I'd try it anyway and I'm so glad I did.'

MALE CONDOM

The latex condom or sheath is 98 per cent effective as a contraceptive when used correctly every time. It is usually obvious if it has broken or slipped off, so you'll know if you need to seek emergency contraception. And it protects against sexually transmitted diseases.

Side effects are rare, unless one of you is allergic to latex. Alternative materials include synthetic rubber, polyurethane or a form of animal tissue known as 'natural skin'. Some condoms contain a spermicidal lubricant, but if this causes a skin reaction there are many other varieties available.

This is a useful method if you know you can always rely on your partner to use it. Many long-term couples use condoms as a harmless alternative to hormonal or intrauterine contraception.

▶ *Polyurethane and natural skin condoms are not strong enough to protect against the transmission of sexual diseases.*

▶ *If you suffer from menopausal vaginal dryness, it's even more important to use a condom during non-monogamous sex, as damaged skin increases your risk of infection.*

FEMALE CONDOM – THE FEMIDOM

A female version of the condom, the Femidom is a fine polyurethane sheath that slips into the vagina and covers the vulva. It is 95 per cent effective as a contraceptive, when a fresh Femidom is used correctly every time. Importantly, it also prevents transmission of sexual infections.

You need to insert it before your partner's penis comes in contact with the area. You place the closed end in your vagina, holding the soft inner ring between your finger and thumb. Then push the Femidom as far up the vagina as possible, making sure the outer ring stays outside. Make sure that the penis enters the vagina inside the condom, not between the condom and the vaginal wall. You may need to hold it in place during sex to stop it being pushed inside. Afterwards, you have to twist the outer ring to keep the semen inside and gently pull the Femidom out, then wrap it up and drop it in a bin.

▶ *The female condom may suit you if you're a confident woman who isn't currently in a relationship and who only needs occasional contraception. You should be careful not to risk infection with HIV or other sexually transmitted diseases.*
▶ *This method will not suit anyone who feels inhibited about putting a Femidom in.*
▶ *If you feel comfortable with inserting a Femidom, you have a method that combines health protection with contraception and has no side effects or long-term risks.*

Top tip
Regardless of what contraception you are using, you must use a condom (male or female) if you have any sexual contact with someone whose sexual-health status you do not know for certain.

DIAPHRAGM AND CERVICAL CAP

The diaphragm is a rubber cup that you insert deep into your vagina each time before you have intercourse. The cervical cap is a smaller version that fits snugly over the cervix. Both have to be used with spermicide, and are then between 92 per cent and 96 per cent effective as contraceptives.

These methods can be put in before you meet your partner and are not usually detectable.

▶ *The diaphragm and the cap are harmless, non-hormonal and you're in control.*
▶ *Unlike condoms, neither the diaphragm nor the cap can prevent transmission of infections.*

NATURAL FAMILY PLANNING

You can reduce the likelihood of pregnancy by working out when you are going to ovulate. This involves making daily observations of your temperature and cervical secretions to calculate the eight or nine days when you are most fertile. If you do this correctly, family-planning experts say, it can be highly successful. But you have to be very organized and remember to fill in your chart every day.

You can back this method up with fertility measuring devices, available from pharmacies. The best known of these devices in the UK, Persona, is a handheld computerized monitor used with a set of urine-test sticks to measure your hormonal levels. The computer interprets the changing levels to predict ovulation. Used correctly, it is 94 per cent effective.

As it uses no drugs or devices, there are no risks (other than of pregnancy) and no side effects. You can either abstain from sex during your fertile period or use other methods such as condoms. It's useful if you're not too worried about becoming pregnant, but generally better for spacing out your family.

It's difficult to make natural family planning work if you're not in a steady relationship, and it almost rules out spontaneity with a new partner.

▶ *Predicting your ovulation is more complicated when your periods have become irregular.*
▶ *This method is not recommended during the perimenopause unless you know you would be prepared to go through with either an abortion or an unplanned pregnancy. The risk of birth defects and pregnancy complications is higher at this age.*

STERILIZATION

This is one of the most popular forms of contraception in the UK, where it is used by about a quarter of all couples. Both male and female sterilization are almost 100 per cent effective.

Male sterilization, or vasectomy, is a simple operation carrying very few risks. It does not reduce men's sex drive.

Insight

Fears raised a few years ago about male sterilization causing prostate cancer turned out to be unfounded.

Female sterilization, or tubal ligation, is a bigger operation, usually done under general anaesthetic and with a small risk of internal bleeding. It involves cutting or blocking the fallopian tubes, through which eggs move from the ovaries to the uterus. Although theoretically reversible, the chances of success are much lower than for a man, especially for a woman of perimenopausal age. On the other hand, in very rare cases the fallopian tubes mend themselves.

▶ *Sterilization is useful to put an end to contraceptive worries if you're in a long-term stable relationship, or if you're certain you won't want any more children even with a new partner.*
▶ *Female sterilization isn't the same as a hysterectomy, and won't cause early menopause or premature ageing.*

Emergency contraception

Many women change their form of contraception for health reasons during their forties. This is a sensible move, and barrier methods have a very high success rate once you get used to them. But there's a downside to swapping from an almost fail-safe method such as the Pill. When you're dealing with condoms for the first time in 20 years, you may make a mistake or even forget to use one.

If you have had unprotected intercourse, or used a barrier method that didn't work, such as a split condom, you can now buy emergency contraception over the counter in pharmacies. It is also available from sexual-health clinics and GPs who deal with contraception. Not all GPs do, so check before making an appointment.

The special progestogen-only Pill has an 84 per cent success rate if you take it within 72 hours of unprotected intercourse. That's much less effective than the regular Pill, but not much worse than some other forms of contraceptive. Taken between 72 and 120 hours later, it may still work, but the success rate is only about 63 per cent.

Although some people call this abortion, it is in fact contraception. Abortion can only take place after a fertilized egg has been implanted in the womb. The exact working of the 'morning-after pill' isn't known for certain. It may stop an egg being implanted, or it may work by preventing or delaying ovulation, so no egg is even fertilized.

Another option is to have an emergency IUD implanted. This is almost guaranteed to prevent pregnancy, if you have it put in within five days of unprotected intercourse. It is also claimed to be 99 per cent effective if inserted within five days after you ovulated – but that's difficult to predict during the perimenopause, when ovulation may have become irregular. It won't be inserted more than five days after you would have ovulated, as it would cause miscarriage if you were pregnant.

The menopause and the Pill

If you're not on the Pill, changes to your menstrual cycle give an early sign of approaching perimenopause. Your periods may become irregular as you start ovulating less frequently. Your bleeding may become lighter, or in some cases heavier. At this time, too, some women develop premenstrual syndrome (PMS) with mood swings, anxiety or depression just before a period starts.

When you're taking the combined Pill, however, the monthly bleeds are not real periods, as you are not ovulating. They are withdrawal bleeds, as the progestogen component of the pill makes your womb slough off the lining that has developed while you were taking the oestrogen. So you continue the monthly bleeds as long as you stay on the Pill.

Meanwhile, the oestrogen you are taking works like HRT, controlling some of the most noticeable symptoms of the menopause, such as the vasomotor symptoms of hot flushes and night sweats. So you probably won't know your perimenopause has started.

On the progestogen-only Pill (POP), you are not taking any oestrogen, so you will encounter the menopausal symptoms that are caused by oestrogen withdrawal.

Your doctor can take blood tests to check the levels of circulating hormones. Low oestrogen and high follicle-stimulating hormone (FSH) levels are taken as a sign that perimenopause has started. But these results can vary enormously, even within the same day, and you may get normal readings when you've actually started the perimenopause. They don't tell you exactly how far along you have progressed and can't be relied on for certainty. FSH levels are a particularly unreliable indicator of perimenopause when you're on the combined Pill.

Tests should be done on the last day of your pill-free phase. But if it's really important to know for certain, consider coming off the

Pill for a few months and using barrier methods of contraception instead. Tests taken after a few months off the combined Pill may be more accurate. They should be repeated after another two months anyway, to check whether FSH readings are still high.

Doctors now recommend stopping any kind of hormonal contraception when you reach 55.

If my periods stop and I'm not pregnant, am I perimenopausal?

Bear in mind that if you stop taking the Pill in your thirties or forties, it can take months for your menstrual cycle to re-establish itself. Meanwhile, if you have hormone tests during this time, the results may suggest that you have started the perimenopause. In reality, your body may just be taking its time to start ovulating again. So give yourself time, and make sure your diet and lifestyle are supporting your reproductive system.

You may also stop having periods for other reasons that aren't connected with the menopause.

Your body needs a certain amount of fat to support vital functions. If your weight falls below a safe level, it will start to jettison functions that aren't essential to survival. Reproduction is one of the first to go, as it is not only non-essential, but would put a further strain on your body. So don't go on stringent diets or let your body weight fall too low.

Check your body mass index (BMI) at http://tinyurl.com/7yqp3: it should not be below 19. If you are just a little above this but not ovulating, your weight might still be too low for your personal metabolism, so try eating some more healthy carbohydrates, such as baked potatoes and plenty of fruit.

Excessive exercise can disrupt the menstrual cycle too, even if your weight doesn't fall below a safe limit.

A sudden shock to the system can stop ovulation for a few months. This can be either an emotional shock such as a relationship break-up, or a physical shock such as an illness or major operation.

Loss of periods can also be a sign of something wrong with the hormones, not only reproductive hormones but also those produced by the pituitary, thyroid or adrenal glands.

You should consult your doctor if you stop having periods at any time when you're not pregnant.

I want a baby

Women's fertility declines steeply after the mid-thirties. If you are past 35 and considering having a baby, now is the time to make up your mind. Don't rely on still being fertile even in your early forties. It becomes more difficult to carry a baby to term: a quarter of all confirmed pregnancies end in miscarriage after the age of 40.

Insight

Most women's fertility starts declining sharply in the late thirties. But our bodies age at very different rates. The variation is caused by genetics, but also affected by our health, lifestyles and even things that happened to us in the womb. So you can't presume you – or your partner – still have a few years of fertility left.

If you aren't sure if you have started the perimenopause, you can take hormone tests. But don't rely too much on the results, as hormone levels can be erratic and misleading during the perimenopause.

If you are trying unsuccessfully for a baby, find out if you need to make any lifestyle changes or have a health condition that can easily be treated. Start making enquiries about assisted fertility at the same time: waiting lists are long and time is not on your side.

Making some healthy changes in your lifestyle may improve your chance of a successful pregnancy.

If you're above a certain weight you may also have difficulty conceiving even if you are ovulating. Women whose body mass index is above BMI 30, and who are therefore considered 'obese', have a much lower success rate with fertility treatment. For every extra point above BMI 30, researchers have found a four per cent fall in success rates compared with women who are simply overweight (BMI 25–9).

Being underweight is even more likely to stop you conceiving, as you may not be ovulating at all.

- ▶ *Take some exercise most days, but don't overdo it as this can suppress ovulation.*
- ▶ *Eat healthily, with plenty of fresh fruit and vegetables.*
- ▶ *If you are overweight, try to slim down at a gentle pace. Stringent dieting can also prevent ovulation.*
- ▶ *Don't smoke or take any other unnecessary drug.*

Insight

We are now so used to the message about fertility declining during the thirties, that many women think pregnancy is unlikely after that. That's probably why sexual-health workers in the UK report an increase in the number of unplanned pregnancies among women over 40. Be warned!

Summary

If your periods stop after you turn 50, you need to continue using contraception for a year after the final period. If they stop before you're 50, continue for two years to be on the safe side. If you're on the combined Pill, you should swap to another method at 50, but on the progestogen-only Pill you can continue until you are 55. If you're using hormonal contraception or HRT and don't know when your periods would have stopped, continue using some form of contraception until you're 55.

Always use a male or female condom (whether or not you are using other contraception) with anyone whose sexual-health status you do not know for certain.

If you've been using the same form of contraception for years, it may no longer be the safest and most effective for you, especially if you've put on weight.

Although your fertility starts declining in your late thirties, you can still get pregnant into your fifties. If you are trying for a baby, lifestyle changes may help you conceive.

Action plan: finding the right contraception or maximizing fertility

1 *Your contraceptive needs may change during your forties, so make an appointment with your well-woman clinic or family-planning nurse to find out what is available.*
2 *Considering your present lifestyle, look at the latest options and see if anything would suit you better.*
3 *If you are on the combined Pill and wish to continue, but your doctor recommends coming off it, ask the reasons why. It may be that a small lifestyle change such as losing weight or giving up smoking would put you back in the safe category.*
4 *If you are trying for a baby, make any lifestyle changes that may help. Start enquiring about assisted reproduction options at the same time, even if you're hoping not to need them, as the process can take a long time.*

10 THINGS TO REMEMBER

1   After about 35, it's an idea to review your method of contraception, especially if you're on the Pill, as your risk factors will be changing.

2   Advances in the past few years may have made a different form of contraception more suitable for you.

3   The combined oral contraceptive Pill (COC) increases your risk of blood clots and stroke.

4   If you have risk factors such as being overweight or smoking, you'll be advised not to continue the combined oral contraceptive (COC) after your mid-thirties. If you're not at high risk, you can stay on it until you're 50.

5   The oestrogen in a COC works like HRT, controlling menopausal symptoms such as hot flushes.

6   The progestogen-only Pill (POP) is considered safe to take at any age. It has different side effects from the COC, and has to be taken at the same time every day without fail.

7   The intrauterine system (IUS) is a modern take on the (non-hormonal) intrauterine contraceptive device. Containing progestogen, the IUS can reduce the pain and blood loss of heavy periods.

8   There are several other forms of contraception that have no side effects and are still well over 90 per cent effective.

9   Fertility declines sharply from your late thirties on, although you can still become pregnant in your fifties.

10 If you still plan to have children, remember that it's not just about getting pregnant. Miscarriage also becomes much more likely after the late thirties.

7

. . . .

Sexuality

In this chapter you will learn:
- *why you may lose some interest in sex at this time*
- *what you can do about this, if you wish to*
- *the facts about remedies advertised on the Internet*
- *how to combat urogenital symptoms caused by loss of oestrogen.*

Some women lose a lot of their libido, or sex drive, as they go through the menopause. Others still have their libido, but find that hormonal changes make sex difficult or uncomfortable. Some women also encounter problems with the genital area: infections such as thrush or cystitis, itchy discomfort or even urinary incontinence.

All of these problems are connected with the hormonal changes we go through during this time. As the body's production of oestrogen slows down, skin becomes thinner and dryer. This affects the genital area more than most, because skin is already sensitive there. The vagina shrinks a little, becoming shorter and narrower. The skin there and on the area just outside, the vulva, becomes more fragile – and damaged skin is vulnerable to infections. The drying effect reduces the secretions that gently bathe the area to keep it healthy. And when you're sexually aroused, lubrication is slower and less abundant than in the past.

The loss of oestrogen also weakens inner muscles, including those that hold back the flow of urine. For many women, the worst symptom of menopause is urinary incontinence. This can take the form of either stress incontinence, when sneezing or laughing makes you lose some urine, or urge incontinence, when you just can't get to the loo in time.

These issues can all be sorted out, with or without the use of HRT or other medicines. Although a lot of the treatment is self-help, the information in this chapter is just guidance. It's best to see a doctor, or a specialist nurse, who can provide individual advice and teach you how to do the relevant exercises.

Loss of libido

This is a busy time in many women's lives, when sex can take a back seat. Sheer exhaustion is a major reason to lose interest in sex at any age – your need for sleep is more powerful. Stress attacks the libido in other ways, preventing you from relaxing into this familiar rhythm. And depression can take all the joy out of any activity, killing your appetite for pleasure. All these factors are problems in themselves. Advice given in Chapters 4, 11 and 13 on mind and mood, lifestyle and fitness is aimed at tackling them, which could be enough to revive your libido at the same time.

Sometimes it's just that the spark has gone out of a long-term relationship. Especially if your lives revolve around children, you may have slipped into seeing each other as Mum and Dad – friendly, even loving, but not at all sexual.

Insight

Loss of libido is a side effect of some drugs, including SSRI (selective serotonin reuptake inhibitor) antidepressants. Never give up antidepressants abruptly, though, as this can cause dangerous mental disturbances.

All kinds of psychological pressures can also crush the playful, passionate side of your nature, including hang-ups about your (or your partner's!) ageing body, and discomfort caused by weight gain or other midlife changes. Concern and anxiety about bladder weakness, common at this time, is enough to put some women off the very idea of sexual intimacy, especially with a new partner.

WHAT'S NORMAL?

People selling 'remedies' for loss of interest in sex give it names such as female sexual arousal disorder (FSAD), female sexual dysfunction (FSD) or hypoactive sexual desire disorder (HSDD). This is one of the 'medicalized conditions' that provoked the *British Medical Journal* to castigate drug companies for making healthy people think they're ill. Some practitioners say that a loss of libido should be treated if the woman feels distressed by it. But who wouldn't be distressed by thinking they're ill or abnormal?

What if our highly sexualized world reflects only the interests of young male consumers, blown up to giant size by the companies that advertise to them? One influential study reported that 43 per cent of women aged 18–59 have 'female sexual dysfunction'. But if nearly half the female population are less interested in sex than they're supposed to be, doesn't that mean researchers are mistaken about what's normal?

For many women, the menopause provides new opportunities to put their energy into interests they didn't have time for before. If they're happily single, losing interest in sex isn't a problem. The same is true if they're in a low-sex or no-sex relationship – and these are more common than we're led to believe. In some societies, this is a time of life when both sexes are expected to develop more spiritual concerns.

Relaxed and satisfied

'There is the relief of not having to worry about pregnancy even though the libido is satisfied with less, sexually, rather than more,' says Christine. 'Perhaps, now in my fifties I am more relaxed about my life. I was also ready to find the man I wanted to marry – and did.'

Bringing your libido back to life

A lack of libido becomes a problem if you want a more active sex life, or if it's damaging your relationship with a partner.

Sometimes the problem is that vaginal drying has made sex difficult and painful. This is a direct result of loss of oestrogen, and it's one of the cases where HRT can help. You don't even need to take pills: oestrogen can be delivered via creams, pessaries or tablets that you insert into your vagina, or a ring that stays inside. Taking oestrogen alone can cause cancer of the womb lining, so it's usually prescribed with progestogen, which has a protective effect. But if the oestrogen dose in a vaginal product is low enough, you don't even need to take progestogen. If you've had a hysterectomy, you don't need progestogen anyway.

The downside is that the symptoms return when you stop taking the HRT. And some experts find that, after your body has adapted to using replacement oestrogen, the symptoms are more severe when it's withdrawn. HRT can also cause symptoms such as bleeding and breast tenderness.

It's not only about dryness, though. What if you've just lost interest? There are both drug and herbal remedies available that promise to rekindle women's sex drive. Some, such as testosterone, are available from a doctor, in some countries at least. But most are bought on the Internet, where they are widely advertised. Read on to find out the facts about them before buying.

Insight

Drugs and other treatments aimed at reviving women's sex drive, for example through increasing blood flow to the genital area, have not proved very effective. Experts suggest this is because they are too simplistic, and that women's libido involves psychological and emotional factors too.

TAKING TESTOSTERONE

Although testosterone is described as a 'male hormone', women also make small amounts of it, and it contributes to our sexual drive. The ovaries go on producing a little even after the menopause, but women who have had their ovaries removed may feel a loss of libido for this reason.

Insight

A woman who has had a hysterectomy may feel a loss of libido due to lack of testosterone, even if her ovaries were not removed, as their blood supply may have been reduced by the operation.

Testosterone therapy may increase women's libido after menopause, and especially after a hysterectomy. However, studies have shown that a woman's libido isn't related to the amount of testosterone, or other hormones, measurable in her blood. This may be partly because women's sensitivity to their hormones varies enormously, from one individual to another.

Although studies of testosterone therapy haven't shown any serious side effects, the volunteers were only taking it for a few months. Long-term effects may include deepening of the voice, excess hair growth and other de-feminizing features. Although used in the UK, the testosterone patch was denied a licence by the US Food & Drug Administration because of concerns about these and other possible, as yet unknown, long-term effects.

OTHER DRUGS

Sildenafil (Viagra), tadalafil (Cialis) and vardenafil (Levitra) are used to help men get erections. They may also cause numerous side effects including dizziness, nausea and heart attack. They're not licensed for use by women, but some women have tried them.

In medical research, these and similar drugs have been found to stimulate blood flow to a woman's vulva and increase lubrication. But this doesn't solve the problem of a low libido for women. Women's libido is very much less genitally focused than men's. The drugs have little or no effect on a woman's libido, as they don't affect the brain.

Several drugs are being developed to try to address a lack of libido in women, including a new testosterone gel and a drug to act on serotonin receptors in the brain.

A new selective estrogen/oestrogen receptor modulator (SERM) called Ophena is intended to relieve vaginal dryness. This could help a woman whose libido has been hit by anxiety about painful sex.

HERBAL APHRODISIACS

Herbs that are marketed as aphrodisiacs mainly aim, like drugs, to help men get erections. In some cases they can do this. But, like drugs, they have little or no effect on a woman's libido. And any herbal preparation that can affect sexual functioning is likely to be as strong as a drug, but with less controlled effects.

▶ *Yohimbe* (Pausinystalia yohimbe) *may increase blood circulation and sensitivity in the genital area for both men and women. It also causes a frightening array of side effects including anxiety, tremors, nausea and high blood pressure, and interacts dangerously with numerous medicines including antidepressants.*

▶ *Damiana* (Turnera diffusa) *is promoted as an aphrodisiac, but there's no reliable evidence that it is either effective or safe. It can react with diabetes drugs.*

Insight

There is little evidence for the effectiveness of any herbal aphrodisiacs and many have harmful side effects and drug interactions.

MAKING TIME TO RECONNECT

Often, the problem is compounded by a relationship that has gone flat. In this case, you need to make a decision to reconnect. Good sex doesn't happen in a vacuum, so work on rebuilding the relationship or coaxing it out of a rut. Spend time enjoying each other. Helpful tactics include the following:

▶ *Take a sensual weekend away with your partner at a spa or seaside resort. Shed most of your clothes, rediscover the pleasure of rippling waves or essential oils on your skin, and take that body pleasure back to your hotel room for long and sensuous nights.*

▶ *Schedule a regular evening for relaxing with wine and whatever the two of you find erotic.*

▶ *Browse online catalogues for vibrators and other products that could bring the fun back into your sex life. Some chains of sex shops target female customers these days, and make a point of welcoming women.*

▶ *Good sex doesn't have to be penetrative genital sex. Discover the pleasures of hands, tongues and every part of your body.*

▶ *Get back into the habit of sharing everyday, non-erotic pleasures too.*

▶ *Most importantly of all, give yourselves time. Long, slow foreplay is not only helpful to allow your body time to produce lubrication and make your vagina a welcoming environment, it's also at the heart of good sex, for both partners.*

LUBRICANTS

Many non-hormonal products can help to lubricate the vagina and vulva. Look at a pharmacist's shelves or reputable online companies' websites for a range of different options. Water-based gels (safe for use with condoms) include KY-Jelly, Senselle, Sensilube, Wet, Vielle, Astro-glide, Forplay, Liquid Silk, Eros Woman.

Numerous other products have slightly different formulations to be denser, lighter, flavourless or whatever else you want. Some contain extra ingredients such as menthol derivates for a mild tingle, bringing extra blood to the area.

These products are for use purely as lubricants during love-making. Other products aim to keep the area healthy by preventing, or slowing down, the loss of moisture and resilience in the vaginal walls. A soy-based gel called Phyto Soya is claimed to help keep your vaginal walls healthy when used twice a week. It doubles as an effective lubricant when you're making love. Bioadhesive moisturizer gels such as Replens have been found to rehydrate vaginal tissues more effectively than ordinary lubricant. It is available over the counter and on prescription.

Many other lubricants are available at shops or through mail order online. Why not try a selection to see which ones suit you and your partner best?

Top tip

Don't let dryness ruin your sex life when there are many forms of lubricant available. Having sexual intercourse more often increases the body's ability to produce its own lubrication.

Insight

Vaginal dryness is a problem even if you are not sexually active, as it can lead to thrush and cystitis. Vaginal moisturisers, available from chemists over the counter or on prescription, are for regular use regardless of your sex life. They're not the same as lubricants, which are applied before or during sex.

Infections

It's an annoying fact of life that infections become more common as genital skin becomes more fragile. One of the most common is thrush, a yeast infection, usually in the vagina, that causes an itchy, smelly discharge. Another is cystitis, a urinary infection that causes intense burning pain when you pass water. These are not sexually transmitted infections, although sex can encourage them.

Both conditions need medical treatment if they last more than a couple of days, as they can spread inwards. This is particularly important with cystitis, which can lead on to more serious bladder infections and inflammation.

Don't take it for granted that these are just part of the menopause. If you're getting frequent infections, ask your doctor to check they don't stem from any other cause. Frequent bouts of thrush, for example, can be a sign of diabetes.

Reduce the risk of cystitis and thrush by:

▸ *wearing loose cotton clothes*
▸ *showering rather than taking long hot baths*
▸ *never using chemicals in the genital area, especially douches or 'vaginal cleansers' – warm water and mild soap are all you need.*

Top tip

You become more susceptible to sexual infections as you grow older, because your skin tears more easily. So be even more careful to use condoms with a new partner. And always use water-based lubricants, as oil-based lubricants damage condoms.

▶ *Yogurt can be applied to the vulva and vagina to soothe the itching of thrush. It may also counteract the bacterial infection.*

▶ *A dilution of one part cider vinegar, to seven parts water dabbed on the area with cotton wool, is a folk remedy for thrush. It is intended to restore a healthier balance of acid to alkali.*

▶ *Pouring a pint of boiling water over a teaspoonful of cherry stalks makes an infusion that, strained and drunk lukewarm, can help relieve the burning pain of cystitis. Drink as much as you can, up to three litres a day, to flush the infection out.*

▶ *Cranberry juice discourages bacteria from sticking to the bladder wall.*

If any of these remedies don't work within a few days, or the pain becomes unbearable, see your doctor for a prescription. If you are given antibiotics, eating plenty of yogurt may help preserve the good bacteria in your digestive system.

Urinary incontinence

The decline in oestrogen production also affects your bladder, making urinary incontinence a dispiriting side effect of menopause for many women. Fear of losing bladder control during sex makes some women lose self-confidence and avoid sexual intimacy.

Losing a few drops of urine comes as a shock to women during the menopause, if they've never encountered it before. Those who have had children may well remember this from the past, and know that, once again, the problem can be solved.

Self-help techniques are frequently taught by doctors or specialists, because they have been proved effective. Kegel exercises (see below) are most useful with stress incontinence, which is the most common kind at menopause. As a bonus, the exercises strengthen the grip of your vagina. This alone can bring a new buzz to your sex life, increasing enjoyment for both you and your partner.

Bladder retraining may be taught for urge incontinence, which is more likely to stem from bladder infections.

There are numerous products that help with urinary incontinence, such as devices that fit in the vagina and encourage the urethra back into place. HRT may help, and there are medicines called anticholinergics that soothe an overactive bladder.

If all else fails, there are several small surgical procedures that can cure the problem.

To relieve urinary incontinence:

▶ *eat plenty of fruit and vegetables and drink enough fluids to prevent constipation, which puts more pressure on the bladder*
▶ *avoid caffeine, fizzy drinks, alcohol and anything else that can irritate the bladder*
▶ *don't do strenuous work or heavy lifting*
▶ *take regular exercise, such as walking*
▶ *always empty your bladder before making love.*

Top tip

If you are overweight, losing some weight could ease your incontinence by taking pressure off the pelvic floor.

Special exercises such as Kegel (see next page) teach you how to rebuild the strength of your pelvic floor, to prevent any extra pressure on the bladder. Latest research has shown that the exercises work better than any other treatment, including HRT and surgery.

For Kegel exercises, you need to isolate the right muscles to work on, which isn't always easy. If you've got it right, following the instructions in this chapter should bring

(Contd)

an improvement within a few weeks. But if you've tried unsuccessfully for a couple of months, don't give up. The exercises really work once you're doing them correctly. Ask at your doctor's surgery or well-woman clinic for help from a specially trained nurse or physiotherapist.

KEGEL EXERCISES

1 *While using the loo, stop the flow of urine, let it start again and stop it again. Don't do this as an exercise, because it can irritate the bladder – only do it if you need to re-check that you're exercising the right muscles.*
2 *Hold in your anal muscles as if stopping yourself passing wind. Release and tighten again to get the feel of this set of muscles.*
3 *Put a finger flat on the perineum (the skin between the vagina and the anus) and squeeze your muscles as if stopping yourself urinating. Then tighten muscles as if to stop yourself passing wind. Try to feel the pelvic floor lifting itself a tiny distance up, towards your head. Your finger should feel the tiny lifting movement inside.*
4 *Ensure you're lifting muscles in and up. Rest a hand on your lower abdomen: if this pushes against your hand when you make the effort, you're straining downwards instead.*
5 *Make sure you're not using other muscles. Relax your buttocks, thighs and abdominal muscles. Don't hold your breath.*
6 *Hold the lift for four seconds, relax for four seconds, and repeat ten to 15 times. Work up gradually to holding for ten seconds at a time.*
7 *Do the exercises for at least five minutes, three times a day, preferably in different positions: lying, sitting and standing.*

Summary

Many women find their sex drive dwindling as they go through the perimenopause. Shortage of hormones, especially oestrogen and to a lesser extent testosterone, can reduce libido. It also makes the skin around the genital area dry and fragile, and therefore susceptible to infections. It also weakens internal muscles, which can lead to urinary incontinence. But much can be done to improve the situation: numerous self-help techniques can reduce the risk of infections and targeted exercises can restore bladder control.

HRT may help improve skin strength and moisture and, along with various other drugs, has been put forward to reverse loss of libido. But as menopausal loss of libido stems from psychological and practical factors as well as hormonal changes, it responds best to a blend of efforts – including allowing yourself more time to enjoy sex.

Action plan: restoring pleasure in your body

1 *If you suffer from urinary incontinence, frequent urogenital infections, painful sex or loss of libido, see your doctor to check that nothing else is causing the problem.*
2 *With other causes ruled out, try the relevant self-help techniques described in this chapter.*
3 *If self-help techniques don't start helping within a few weeks, ask your doctor for further advice.*
4 *If you're offered drugs, check to ensure the side effects aren't likely to be worse than your present conditions.*
5 *Give yourself and your partner time together to reconnect with each other. Relax and enjoy the process of rebuilding an intimate relationship that may have been sidelined in recent years.*

10 THINGS TO REMEMBER

1 As oestrogen levels decline in the later stages of perimenopause, women often lose some of their sex drive.

2 Loss of libido is also a side effect of some drugs, including selective serotonin reuptake inhibitor (SSRI) antidepressants.

3 Oestrogen nourishes skin and membranes. As the body's production falls, the vaginal walls become dryer, less flexible and more easily damaged.

4 Vaginal dryness not only makes intercourse painful but can lead to infections such as thrush and cystitis.

5 Low oestrogen levels can also weaken internal muscles, which may lead to urinary incontinence.

6 There are numerous products that prevent vaginal dryness, including moisturisers and oestrogen creams.

7 Use of lubricants is part of many couples' foreplay, and there's an ever-increasing range of options on sale.

8 Special exercises can tone up internal muscles, improving vaginal grip as well as bladder control.

9 If those don't work, hospital specialists have many more options, from techniques you can learn to minor operations.

10 The best sex aid in midlife is time. Take time to reconnect with yourself and your partner and give your libido a chance to come back to life.

8

Hormone replacement therapy

In this chapter you will learn:
- *the facts behind HRT health scares*
- *what conditions HRT can help with*
- *how to choose the form that works best for you*
- *ways to use HRT for the best possible effects, with the least harm to your health.*

The big question facing women as they approach the menopause is whether or not to take hormone replacement therapy (HRT). Even those who don't encounter any problems during this transition may wonder if it's worth taking hormones to reduce their risk, in later life, of suffering conditions such as osteoporosis or heart disease.

But the evidence, and resulting medical advice, keeps changing. What has led up to this? And how do we know who's giving us the best information?

Hopes and shocks

Fifty years ago, doctors thought they had discovered a medicine that could practically stop the ageing process, for women at least. Treatment with oestrogen was not only thought to cure the symptoms of menopause, it was also believed to protect against the diseases of old age and allow women to keep their youthful looks and figures. Books published in the 1960s promised women that HRT could help them stay 'forever feminine' or avoid the menopause altogether.

The 1970s, however, saw a steep rise in the incidence of uterine (womb) cancer, the most common kind being endometrial cancer, which affects the endometrium or womb lining. Many women died before this was found to stem from the effects of replacement oestrogen. Manufacturers quickly added a new ingredient: progestogen or progestin, a synthetic version of the hormone progesterone. This protected the lining of the uterus, and the number of women taking HRT increased again.

During the 1990s, improvements in formulation tackled some of the side effects that had made women give up on HRT. By the end of the decade, the number of women giving up within the first year had halved.

At the turn of the twenty-first century, up to half of all women in some countries were trying HRT as they reached the menopause. In 2001 HRT was being used by more than 100 million women around the world, including an estimated 1.5 million in Britain. It caught on most in countries where women were already used to taking hormone tablets in the form of the contraceptive Pill.

By this time, reports were suggesting that HRT might do a lot more than just reduce menopausal symptoms and keep women looking young. Reports claimed that HRT might protect women from heart disease, cancers, even Alzheimer's and other dreaded conditions of old age. But some studies were starting to show other effects: HRT was being linked with an increase in other diseases, especially breast cancer.

With so many women taking HRT, several large studies were set up to find out exactly what effects it was having. Two of them in particular were enormous. In Britain, the Million Women Study recruited 1.3 million women aged 50 and upwards between 1996 and 2001: a quarter of the entire female population of that age. And in the United States, the Women's Health Initiative (WHI) recruited 160,000 women for a study starting in 1991.

Insight

The more people that take part in a research study, the more accurate its findings are likely to be. With small numbers, the results can be skewed by chance or coincidence. The Million Women Study, which showed many harmful effects of HRT, actually involved 1.3 million women, so its results are especially convincing.

These large studies started reporting their results in the early 2000s. The results were devastating:

▶ *HRT was found to increase the risk of serious diseases, such as breast cancer and strokes.*
▶ *The expected benefits in preventing conditions such as heart disease and dementia had not materialized.*
▶ *The WHI trials were stopped early because the risk to women's health in continuing was deemed unacceptable.*
▶ *In 2003, a Swedish study was also stopped early, after finding that women who had survived breast cancer were nearly four times more likely to develop another breast tumour if they used HRT.*

When all this bad news was reported, the number of women taking HRT plunged immediately. This was followed a few years later by a drop in the number of new breast cancer cases diagnosed in the USA.

In 2007, a new report from the WHI team led to claims by some HRT supporters that the risks were not as great as originally thought and the drop in breast cancer cases was largely coincidental. This in turn was contradicted by other experts. In 2009, further studies reported that taking combined HRT for five years after menopause doubled the risk of breast cancer, and that women taking HRT were also at higher risk of lung cancer.

THE EVIDENCE IN A NUTSHELL

▶ *HRT reduces the risk of osteoporosis and of cancer of the colon and rectum. Other than that, it has not been shown to reduce the risk of any disease of old age, including dementia.*

▶ *HRT increases the risk of breast cancer, ovarian cancer, blood clots, strokes and gall bladder disease. It also increases the risk of heart disease in older women, though it may not in women who start HRT during the perimenopause.*

▶ *The risk of endometrial cancer is increased by oestrogen therapy but reduced by combined HRT.*

▶ *The increased risk of most of these conditions is fairly small in relation to an average person's overall risk. But because millions of women take HRT, it adds up to large numbers of extra women developing each condition each year.*

▶ *Your personal risk of developing any of these conditions varies enormously according to your individual circumstances and background.*

So the question is whether the risks of taking HRT outweigh the benefits. Every woman's risks and needs are different. If you'd like more detailed information to help you weigh up the evidence, turn to the Appendix.

Meanwhile, millions of women around the world take HRT, and many of them swear by it. Read on to see if it's likely to benefit you.

If they can disagree that much, the benefits can't be overwhelming

'Because both my parents had heart disease, I was quite interested in the possibility of HRT to reduce my risk,' says Julie. 'My periods had started getting lighter, and I was thinking of asking my doctor's advice, more for the long-term benefits than anything else because I wasn't really bothered by any symptoms. Then suddenly it was all-change and HRT wasn't looking quite so good for the heart. I held back from starting it. Then it was definitely harmful, so I was glad I hadn't gone onto it.

'Now you've got people saying "No, it's fine as long as you start it young enough." Well, I'm not any more! And other people are saying "No, it doesn't do any good." It annoys me a bit that we can't get it settled. I think I was right not to go on HRT, because if they can disagree that much about it, the benefits can't be overwhelming.'

Top tip

The amount of information available about HRT can be bewildering. If you screen out all the information that's produced by drug companies, PR firms and industry-funded organizations it becomes a little clearer.

When to use HRT

Women take HRT for many reasons. Because the fine biological tuning of our bodies is so individual, what works for one person may not work for another. Conversely, you may find it has benefits for you that aren't widespread enough to have been validated by researchers.

The two areas where HRT has proved its worth are in:

▶ *controlling the vasomotor symptoms: hot flushes and night sweats*
▶ *relieving urogenital changes: vaginal dryness and urinary problems.*

The vasomotor symptoms of hot flushes and night sweats are what drive most women to take HRT. Thankfully, these rushes of heat should stop within a few weeks, if you're taking the right dose. Some women find them a lot less noticeable within days of starting to take HRT, though others have to persevere for several months.

Urogenital symptoms, such as vaginal dryness, are caused by a general drying of membranes in that area. This dryness can affect the bladder too. As well as making sexual intercourse difficult, it can lead to problems such as thrush and cystitis. This dryness is a direct effect of lack of oestrogen, so HRT can solve this as well. It usually takes a few months to have a noticeable effect, so don't give up before then unless you're getting bad side effects. Some women have persevered for a year and have finally been rewarded with success.

If vaginal dryness is your main symptom, you can often avoid the side effects of systemic HRT – pills or patches that affect the whole body – by using vaginal oestrogen. If you use a low-enough dose to prevent oestrogen entering your bloodstream, you won't need progestogen to protect your womb from cancer. But do discuss this with your doctor first. There are other options too: see Chapter 7 on sexuality.

Most of these symptoms can also be controlled by natural remedies, or by lifestyle changes including healthy diet and exercise. These self-help techniques can even help to relieve hot flushes. It is worth trying these gentle remedies before taking HRT as they have no side effects except a general improvement in health. Whether or not you choose to use HRT too, the lifestyle changes should make your menopause easier.

SYMPTOMS YOU CAN'T STAND

However, some women have symptoms so severe that they can't be controlled without drugs. For them, HRT is worth its weight in gold. Some women have a run of hot flushes that can continue over a period of hours, leaving them weak and drained. Some go months without sleeping well, because they wake up every night drenched in sweat and can't drop off again after showering and changing the sheets. The loss of natural lubrication in your vagina can ruin relationships by making sex painful and difficult. Frequent bouts of thrush can undermine your health, and untreated cystitis can damage the kidneys or bladder.

If you're getting symptoms like these, it's worth trying HRT. If it takes a little longer to work than you expected, do persevere. You may need a higher dose or different drug. And if it causes side effects, ask your doctor about trying a different formulation or product – patches instead of pills, for example.

Some women find their other symptoms are also relieved by HRT. Although there's no scientific evidence to support this, it makes sense if the other problems stemmed from vasomotor or urogenital symptoms.

▶ *Night sweats are a common cause of insomnia during the menopause.*
▶ *Exhaustion caused by severe vasomotor symptoms can make you irritable, unhappy and clumsy. It can even lead to cognitive symptoms: how often have you struggled to find the right word or forgotten to do something, just because you're too tired to think straight?*
▶ *Having hot flushes while you're at work can cause a lot of psychological stress, which may express itself as anxiety or depression.*
▶ *The emotional side effects of vaginal dryness making sex painful and unwelcome are obvious.*

So what you may take for hormonal mood swings could be a natural result of these other symptoms.

However, problems that don't stem from vasomotor or urogenital changes are not usually improved by HRT. If you're suffering from insomnia, heavy bleeding, mood swings or other symptoms, without hot flushes, other remedies (including lifestyle changes) are more likely to help. And if vaginal dryness is your main problem, there are many products available now to relieve it without drugs.

....
Insight

Women's bodies have a very individual response to hormones – both their own and those taken as pharmaceuticals. This is

(Contd)

probably why some women have found HRT helpful with a range of perimenopausal symptoms, even where these haven't been backed by research evidence.

In the end, it's a question of weighing the benefits you're getting right now against the side effects and any long-term risks. If hot flushes are making your life hell, and you can't control them any other way, you may well choose a comfortable life today and leave the future to look after itself.

Any side effects were worth it

'I went to my doctor because I was having up to a dozen hot flushes a day, really violent ones that left me red in the face and drenched in sweat,' says Ursula, an advertising executive. 'I came to hate going out. People could hardly pretend they hadn't noticed! And I worked in a cut-throat office where I felt as if this visible sign of ageing was marking me out for the next job to be cut. I know I should have tried self-help things like meditation but I always felt too stressed to settle down to it.

'HRT made me feel awful at first, like the worst PMS I'd ever had, but it put an end to the hot flushes. I would have thought any side effects, and any long-term effects, were worth it for that alone. After a while I felt confident enough to start trying different prescriptions and eventually got rid of most of the side effects. I dread coming off HRT, in case the hot flushes return.'

Top tip
Remember that HRT does not work as a contraceptive!

HRT options

There's a huge range of choices. Having seen many women trying HRT products, some doctors prefer one sort to another. But if your prescription doesn't suit you, do discuss other options with your doctor.

▶ **Combined HRT** *is the most widely used form of hormone replacement. This includes both oestrogen and progestogen, a synthetic version of the hormone progesterone. The progestogen is necessary to protect the womb lining, which is naturally shed and renewed every month when you're still having periods. There are natural forms of progesterone available, but oddly enough, the body finds them harder to use.*

Insight

Combined HRT may reduce the risk of endometrial cancer.

▶ **Oestrogen-only HRT** *is available for women who have had a hysterectomy. Oestrogen is what provides most of HRT's beneficial effects. But it is known to cause cancer of the womb, so it should not be used by women who still have their uterus. Women who haven't had a hysterectomy can use an oestrogen-only preparation, as long as they also take some form of progestogen.*
▶ **Cyclical HRT** *means taking the oestrogen component every day, adding progestogen for 10–14 days at the end of the monthly cycle. This will produce a period-like monthly bleed. It is most likely to be prescribed to women early in the perimenopause who are still having quite regular periods.*
▶ **Tricyclical HRT** *reduces the bleeding to once every three months. You take oestrogen every day during that time, plus 14 days of progestogen at the end of the 13-week cycle. It is generally prescribed to women later in the perimenopause, whose periods have become irregular.*

► **Continuous combined HRT** *means taking both oestrogen and progestogen every day. It doesn't produce a regular 'period', although there may be some breakthrough bleeding or spotting. This usually stops within a few months. Continuous HRT is offered to women who have already passed the menopause, meaning that they no longer have periods at all.*

HOW TO USE IT

You can take the oestrogen component of HRT in several different 'delivery systems': pills, skin patches, gels, implants or vaginal rings. Progestogen comes in the form of tablets, vaginal gel or pessaries, or an intrauterine system (IUS) called Mirena (see Chapter 6 on contraception), or included in a combined patch.

Patches and gels work as effectively as pills but with a lower dose, as they don't have to go through your digestive system. For this reason, they may cause fewer side effects. Some evidence suggests they are safer in the long term. One report from the Million Women Study shows that HRT delivered through the skin is less likely to cause gall bladder disease.

► **Combined HRT tablets** *are provided in a calendar pack, like the contraceptive Pill. As long as you remember to take them at the same time every day, they are easy to use and you don't have to work out what you should be taking when. But because your digestive system eliminates most of the drug, the dose you swallow has to be high. For this reason, tablets are most likely to cause side effects such as nausea.*
► **Patches** – *combined or oestrogen-only – are applied once or twice a week to your upper buttock, onto clean skin; any lotions or bath-oil residues will stop them sticking. They provide hormones in a lower dose than the tablets. Putting them in a slightly different spot each time reduces the risk of skin irritation. They can be a nuisance on holiday, when you have to remember to cover them from the sun and take them off temporarily while you swim.*

- ► **Oestrogen gels** *are easy to spread like body lotion on a small area of skin. The gel dries in a few minutes and should be left on for at least an hour before you shower or use body lotion. Like patches, they affect the whole body with a lower dose than in tablets.*
- ► **Vaginal oestrogen products** *can be applied in the form of a cream, a tablet inserted with an applicator, or a pessary which you push in like a non-applicator tampon. If the dose is high enough to control non-vaginal symptoms such as hot flushes, you'll also need to use progestogen unless you've had a hysterectomy.*
- ► **A vaginal ring** *can be inserted and left in place for up to three months. Some women find them hard to get used to, but most say that once you get used to one you can hardly tell it's there. You can take it out before intercourse, but this isn't necessary. Those available at present are oestrogen-only.*
- ► **Oestrogen implants** *can be put into the abdomen or buttock under local anaesthetic. They last up to six months. Like contraceptive implants, the downside is that if you don't get on with them, you need another minor operation to remove them.*
- ► **Low-dose vaginal oestrogen preparations** *offer a useful compromise option for women whose only concern is the urogenital symptoms, such as vaginal dryness and cystitis. They are available as pessaries, creams, applicator tablets, or a vaginal ring. These products can be used in the long term, as the dose is meant to be low enough not to affect any other part of the body. (Make sure you're taking the right sort to use in the long term for urogenital symptoms only, as stronger versions need to be balanced with progestogen tablets.) But you should still have regular check-ups.*
- ► *Your GP may prescribe* **'natural progesterone'** *if you wish to try this. It is manufactured, but in a form that's identical to the human hormone. It is not widely prescribed as it is considered to be less effective than progestogen.*

Top tip

Breakthrough bleeding is common in the first three months of taking continuous combined HRT prescriptions. See your doctor if it happens at any other time.

Side effects

Like any other drug, HRT can cause side effects. Most of the ones you're likely to notice at once are annoying rather than dangerous. But some must not be ignored (see box below).

Sometimes HRT exacerbates the very symptoms it's meant to relieve, such as heavy bleeding or mood swings. And if you start taking combined HRT when your periods have stopped, they will come back, unless you take it without a break. Some women don't mind, but others find this brings back period-related problems they were glad to lose.

There are many formulations and dosages of HRT, so do ask your doctor about trying a different product if side effects are bothering you. Some doctors become attached to one brand, but its general safety and effectiveness are irrelevant if it's not helping you.

Hazard signs

Side effects of HRT can be warnings of a serious disorder. Don't ignore **pain, redness** or **swelling in one leg** – this could be a sign of thrombosis, which is a known risk of oestrogen and can be fatal. It is different from the mild muscle cramps, in both legs, that are a common side effect of HRT. **Sudden chest pain** is equally important. See your doctor or go to the A&E department at hospital at once. And go back to your doctor if you have any **unusual or unexpected bleeding**, especially if your periods had stopped before you started HRT.

WILL I PUT ON WEIGHT?

Some women find they put on weight while taking HRT. Unfortunately, this could be a side effect of the menopause itself rather than of the drugs. Once your periods have stopped, it is very easy to gain weight for a number of reasons (as discussed in Chapter 2 on hormones and Chapter 3 on the physical effects).

Opinion is divided on whether HRT makes you put on weight. Some studies have shown that oestrogen encourages weight gain, but only during the first year of treatment. Some women say the opposite – that by reducing the hormonal changes that lead to weight gain, HRT helps them stay in shape. On the other hand, some women say their weight settled down when they came off HRT. It does tend to cause fluid retention, which can look and feel like weight gain. Either way, you can only try different prescriptions and see for yourself. Meanwhile, if you are putting on weight, try the tips offered in Chapter 12 on nutrition and Chapter 13 on fitness.

HRT made me feel depressed

'I found that HRT made me very depressed,' says Chris. 'Only after I had weaned myself off it did a different doctor tell me that it was a common side effect. Let's face it, HRT is not natural, you have to face up to getting older at some time.'

WHAT'S CAUSING THIS?

Some common side effects can be caused by either oestrogen or progestogen. These include:

- ▶ *blood spotting between periods*
- ▶ *headaches*
- ▶ *fluid retention (bloating)*
- ▶ *breast tenderness*
- ▶ *dry eyes.*

Other side effects may stem from one or other component of HRT. Your doctor may be able to prescribe a different form of either oestrogen or progestogen without necessarily changing the other component if that suits you.

> **Insight**
> You can't always tell what causes a side effect, but those of oestrogen tend to occur at any time during a cycle and clear up within three months; those of progestogen are usually limited to the days you're taking the progestogen, but often continue long term.

Side effects of progestogen include:

▶ *mood swings*
▶ *depression*
▶ *acne*
▶ *backache.*

Side effects of oestrogen include:

▶ *nausea*
▶ *indigestion*
▶ *leg cramps*
▶ *vaginal pain*
▶ *thrush*
▶ *painful periods.*

If you're getting nausea or indigestion but are otherwise happy with the tablets you're on, try taking them with a meal. Stretches and exercises may relieve mild leg cramps.

Sometimes, side effects are caused by the delivery system rather than the drug itself. Those taken by mouth tend to contain higher doses, as they have to go through the digestive system before reaching the spot where they'll work. These are also the products that can affect the liver. Other delivery systems such as patches or creams may have fewer side effects, because they can give the same benefits with a lower dose. On the other hand, some women find these irritate their skin. This may be easily solved by using a different patch or cream. The same applies to vaginal products; women who don't get on with creams or gels often find a vaginal ring more suitable.

▶ *You should see your doctor for a check-up every three to six months while you're on HRT, whether or not you have side effects. Your doctor may take your blood pressure and do a breast check and a pelvic examination.*

▶ *Tell your doctor about anything that's changed or that you've noticed, and jot down beforehand any questions that have come up since your last assessment.*

Drug interactions

Make sure your HRT provider knows about any other medicines you are taking. Drugs for other conditions, such as diabetes or epilepsy, may interact with the HRT. It also interacts with drugs for blood clots or breast cancer, but you're unlikely to be taking HRT if you have had these conditions. Ask your doctor about the risks.

Top tip
Ensure that you are on the lowest dose that controls your symptoms.

Coming off HRT

Some of the symptoms relieved by HRT are caused by fluctuating hormones, including some (though not all) cases of hot flushes. If your natural hormone production has settled down by the time you stop the HRT, you shouldn't notice a lot of withdrawal symptoms. But if the condition was caused mainly by lack of oestrogen – vaginal dryness, for example – it will return when you stop taking the hormones.

You may have rebound symptoms if you stop taking HRT suddenly. Unless you've been told to stop at once for health reasons, it's better to wean yourself off the drugs slowly. Ask your GP for advice on doing this effectively, as it will depend on your individual symptoms and dosage.

If hot flushes and sweats were your main problem, try coming off HRT during the winter, when the outside temperature is a bit more helpful.

Conditions caused by lack of oestrogen are the ones that don't wear off naturally after the menopause. So you should switch to other ways of dealing with them. Numerous creams and gels are available from pharmacies to lubricate the vagina and relieve the discomfort of dry skin.

Top tip

Don't take HRT if you are on the combined Pill. If you're on a progestogen-only pill, you can continue this with oestrogen HRT until the age of 55; the Pill also provides the progestogen needed to counteract the oestrogen in HRT.

What are my personal risks?

You are not advised to take HRT if you:

- ▶ *have high blood pressure, unless you are taking medicine that controls it effectively*
- ▶ *have had a cancer of the breast, ovary or womb*
- ▶ *have had a heart attack, a stroke or a blood clot*
- ▶ *have had liver disease*
- ▶ *have any unexplained bleeding (and please tell your doctor about this whether you want to take HRT or not, as it needs to be diagnosed and treated).*

If you have had liver disease, you shouldn't take HRT tablets, as they can affect the liver. Your doctor may prescribe patches or other non-oral preparations.

Be cautious too if you have ever had gall bladder disease, migraines or any of the other conditions that can be caused or exacerbated by taking HRT.

Summary

HRT carries the health risks and benefits summarized in this chapter (see Appendix for more detail). Other drugs suggested as alternatives carry risks of their own, some of which may not yet be known. Doctors now advise women to take HRT in the lowest effective dose, for the shortest possible time, preferably for not more than a couple of years. Women who are suffering badly may accept an added risk of, say, breast cancer later in return for relief from menopausal symptoms now.

Doctors now recommend HRT only if you are suffering badly from the specific symptoms it has been shown to help: hot flushes, night sweats, vaginal dryness and urinary problems. If you have other symptoms that stem from these, such as night sweats causing insomnia, or vaginal dryness causing a loss of sex drive, then taking HRT may help with those too. Some people find HRT evens out mood swings, though others say it makes them worse. Apart from the symptoms just mentioned, HRT hasn't been proved to relieve effects of the menopause. For some women, the side effects of HRT outweigh any benefits it may provide.

HRT is available in numerous formulations and delivery systems, so changing from one to another may alleviate side effects. For vaginal and urinary symptoms, you can apply simple oestrogen products to the area.

Action plan: using HRT to your best advantage

1   *Read all the evidence and weigh it up, bearing in mind that a new study doesn't disprove all earlier ones but simply provides some new information. Keep up to date with latest research if you can, noting whether it has been done by drug companies, cancer charities or independent researchers.*

2   *Work out your risk factors for the diseases that HRT can cause, including your family history of illnesses. Write them down in a list.*

3   *Look into self-help techniques and other options, bearing in mind that other drugs have side effects too, and may not be as well studied as HRT.*

4   *Discuss HRT with your doctor and weigh up the health risks before making a decision about trying it. Consider whether you are being badly troubled by hot flushes, night sweats and genital or urinary problems – the symptoms that HRT is good for. If not, it is unlikely to help with your other symptoms.*

5   *If you take HRT, give it long enough to work unless you are getting disruptive side effects. (Be cautious about taking other drugs to control side effects.) If it's not working, return to your doctor and ask about different formulations or delivery systems, such as patches instead of pills. There are numerous ways of taking HRT which suit different women.*

6   *If your main problems are urogenital – such as painful sex, urinary incontinence, thrush or cystitis – ask about using vaginal oestrogen products. In low doses, these protect the genital area without affecting the rest of the body. Unless you have had a hysterectomy, check whether the product is strong enough to require taking progestogen to prevent womb cancer.*

7   *Look out for side effects, especially the dangerous ones: chest pain, swelling or pain in one leg, or unusual bleeding.*

10 THINGS TO REMEMBER

1 HRT is effective in controlling the vasomotor symptoms (hot flushes and night sweats) and the urogenital symptoms (vaginal dryness and bladder weakness). It hasn't been proved effective for anything else.

2 You should ensure that your doctor knows about any health conditions you have had, or that may run in your family (such as breast cancer) before taking HRT.

3 HRT normally contains both oestrogen and progestogen. Like the contraceptive Pill, it is available in many different formulations, delivering different amounts of hormone over different periods of time.

4 It also comes in various delivery systems such as pills, implants, skin patches, gels and creams.

5 Most women who try HRT give it up because of the side effects, which may be caused by either oestrogen or progestogen.

6 Doctors are sometimes reluctant to prescribe different formulations, but a woman who wants to use HRT should have the chance to find one that's suitable among the plethora of products available.

7 In the long term, HRT reduces the risk of osteoporosis and of cancers of the colon and rectum. It has not been shown to reduce the risk of any old-age disease, including dementia.

8 HRT increases the risk of blood clots, strokes, gall-bladder disease and cancers of the breast, ovary and lung.

(Contd)

9 *It also increases the risk of heart disease in women who start it after menopause. It may have better effects if started before menstrual cycles end, but this is not yet known.*

10 *Doctors now recommend only using HRT if you're suffering badly from vasomotor or urogenital symptoms, using the lowest effective dose and not continuing for more than two years.*

9

Other medical help

In this chapter you will learn:
- *what symptoms your doctor can help you tackle without HRT*
- *what you should do about pre-conditions such as pre-osteoporosis*
- *if and when antidepressants can ease your symptoms.*

Hormone replacement therapy (HRT) isn't the medical profession's only answer to hot flushes and the other nuisances of menopause. You may have been told that you should not take HRT because you're in a high-risk group for some of the diseases it can cause, especially cancers. Or you may not wish to take drugs that have such a strong effect on your hormones. Or perhaps you have tried HRT and not found a formulation that suits you.

If you wish to explore any of the medical options, make an appointment with your regular doctor – who knows your background – and let him/her know you'd like time to talk through various options. If you are seeing a doctor who doesn't know all your details, it can be useful to book a double-length appointment so that you have all the time you need.

These days, you're less likely than in the past to be offered a prescription at every visit to your GP's surgery. Doctors do their best to practise 'evidence-based medicine' – finding out what works rather than necessarily what people are used to. They often try to persuade patients to make dietary changes, take regular exercise and get outdoors more. They're not trying to reduce drug bills, they're keeping up with the latest in scientific research, which shows that such simple changes in lifestyle have better effects than most medicines.

Insight
Doctors are increasingly concerned about drug side effects, interactions and limitations.

The menopausal problems for which women most commonly seek help are:

▶ *vasomotor symptoms – hot flushes and night sweats – signs of a faulty thermostat*
▶ *heavy bleeding*
▶ *mood disturbances, mainly depression, anxiety or mood swings*
▶ *urogenital changes including vaginal dryness, urinary incontinence, cystitis and thrush (see Chapter 7 on sexuality).*

HRT alternatives

Several drugs are available to tackle individual symptoms, but until quite recently only hormone replacement aimed to tackle them all. In recent years, some drugs have come onto the market that aim to have a similar effect to HRT, but without the side effects of hormones.

TIBOLONE

Tibolone, marketed under the name Livial, is a synthetic hormone that combines some of the effects of oestrogen, progesterone and testosterone. It's been described as 'the other HRT', because it is prescribed to combat the vasomotor symptoms and vaginal dryness, and to reduce the risk of osteoporosis.

Tibolone has been found to increase the risk of breast and endometrial cancer. The Million Women Study found that women on tibolone were 1.8 times more likely than non-users to develop endometrial cancer, which is more than the risk posed by oestrogen.

> **Insight**
>
> Older women's risk of having a stroke has been found to increase significantly, when taking tibolone to prevent osteoporosis.

SELECTIVE ESTROGEN/OESTROGEN REUPTAKE MODULATORS (SERMS)

SERMs aim to reproduce some of oestrogen's beneficial actions, such as keeping bones strong, without any of the adverse effects, such as increasing the risk of certain cancers. They work by homing in on molecules called oestrogen receptors, which is where oestrogen usually docks. By taking the place of oestrogen, SERMs can also oppose its effects: the breast-cancer drug tamoxifen, for example, is a SERM.

SERMs have different effects and side effects. Most of them lower cholesterol and strengthen bones, but also increase the risk of blood clots. Some SERMs, especially raloxifene, can actually cause hot flushes, making them unpopular among women at menopause.

Because SERMs can be quite accurately targeted, they work on different areas. Those most relevant to women going through the menopause are:

▶ *DT56a (Femarelle or Tofupill) – this is made from soybeans and tackles menopausal symptoms, including hot flushes, as well as strengthening bones. It is claimed not to increase the risk of blood clots.*
▶ *Ospemifene (Ophena) is available in the US and is expected to be available in the UK some time after 2010. It is said to help protect the vagina and vulva from thinning and becoming susceptible to infections.*
▶ *Raloxifene is prescribed to strengthen bones (but can cause hot flushes).*

Vasomotor symptoms

Several drugs are now available that aim to treat hot flushes and night sweats. Most of them were originally developed to treat other, more serious conditions and may have strong side effects.

With such powerful drugs being used to treat a problem that's not life threatening, there's surprisingly little solid evidence about their benefits and side effects. A 2006 study found that only 43 out of thousands of published studies of these drugs even met strict scientific criteria.

▶ *Some of these drugs have side effects such as weight gain and fatigue that may be mistaken for symptoms of the menopause itself.*
▶ *If you notice any of these, do stop taking the drug rather than seeking treatment for effects it probably caused.*

CLONIDINE

Marketed under the names Catapres or Dixarit, clonidine is a drug that's prescribed to treat migraines or high blood pressure. It has also been found to alleviate hot flushes. Its method of action isn't understood, but it may work by blocking signals sent from the brain to the blood vessels.

Although it has been around for a long time, little good-quality research has been done into this use for clonidine. A 1987 study found it up to 80 per cent effective in reducing hot flushes, but only 29 women took part, including 14 who had the placebo, and the researchers used a skin patch which is not available in the UK.

Common side effects include a dry mouth, nausea, drowsiness and dizziness.

GABAPENTIN

This epilepsy drug has been found to relieve hot flushes. It may also reduce menopausal aches and pains.

However, its side effects include dizziness, tremor, clumsiness, fatigue and weight gain.

Insight

Certain drugs have side effects that may be mistaken for menopausal symptoms themselves. These may include weight gain, fatigue and even hot flushes. If you notice any of these, speak to your doctor about giving up the drug and seeing if the 'symptoms' disappear.

ANTIDEPRESSANTS

Selective serotonin reuptake inhibitors (SSRIs) and serotonin and noradrenaline reuptake inhibitors (SNRIs) are types of antidepressant, including venlafaxine (Efexor), fluoxetine (Prozac) and paroxetine (Seroxat, Paxil).

There's some evidence that they can help to reduce vasomotor symptoms of the menopause and control mood swings. But, as with much research about antidepressants, the results are mixed. They have only been proved effective in short trials, whereas most women seek long-term relief.

SSRIs and SNRIs have numerous unintended effects on both mind and body. People often stop taking them because of immediate side effects such as nausea or agitation. Common long-term side effects include sleep disorders, loss of libido, memory loss and weight gain. And recent research has found that they increase the risk of having a stroke in women over 50. However, some women do find them helpful.

Heavy bleeding

Periods are considered 'heavy' if you're bleeding steadily for more than eight days, losing clots of blood on more than a couple of days, flooding through tampons or pads, or becoming anaemic. However, the main concern is if they are heavy by your personal standards. You may not be losing more than average, but if it's more than you've been used to, and it's bothering you, you should see your doctor.

It is also necessary to check whether heavy bleeding is a sign of menopause, or one of the other conditions that become more common after the age of 40. These conditions include endometriosis, fibroids, polyps, cysts or other changes to the womb and its lining. Most of these are only a problem if they're causing you pain or excessive blood loss. But it might also be an early sign of cancer, so it's worth checking immediately.

You're likely to be given a blood test to see if the loss of iron (which is carried in the bloodstream) has made you anaemic. If so, you may be offered iron supplements. Read Chapter 12 on nutrition for ways to increase it in your diet too.

You should also have a pelvic examination. If your doctor still has questions, you may be referred for investigations such as a biopsy, in which a tiny piece of tissue is removed for analysis; or an ultrasound scan, which shows moving pictures of your internal organs on a screen; or a hysteroscopy, in which a tiny camera is passed into your womb.

Doctors can offer several treatments to help reduce heavy bleeding, including contraceptives, medicines or surgery.

If your bleeding pattern changes suddenly, or you start bleeding again after your periods have stopped, please see your doctor as soon as possible. Many conditions can be successfully treated if diagnosed promptly.

COMBINED CONTRACEPTIVE PILL

This solves the problem of heavy bleeding and period pain for many women. You may need to try different formulations and delivery systems (such as pills or patches) to find the one that's right for you. But because of its oestrogen content, the combined Pill is not suitable for some women. (There is more about this in Chapter 6 on contraception.)

If you are over the age of 35, you'd be advised not to take the combined Pill if you smoke or are overweight. And doctors now recommend that you stop taking the Pill at the age of 50, even if you're in good health.

LEVONORGESTREL INTRAUTERINE SYSTEM (IUS)

Women with heavy periods wouldn't usually consider an intrauterine contraceptive device, as the ordinary kind would make matters worse.

But the levonorgestrel IUS, or Mirena, contains a form of progestogen that is released slowly into the body, preventing the womb lining from building up. This means the womb lining doesn't have to be shed with a monthly or three-monthly bleed. It can be used to bring heavy bleeding under control, and often stops periods altogether.

Side effects may include acne, headaches and breast tenderness.

OTHER DRUGS

Tranexamic acid is a drug that helps blood to clot, and has been found useful in controlling heavy periods. It occasionally causes indigestion, diarrhoea or headaches, but side effects are rare.

Non-steroidal anti-inflammatory drugs (NSAIDs), widely known for their use as painkillers, can also help. They work by reducing the body's production of a hormone-like substance called prostaglandin, which is linked to heavy periods.

Tranexamic acid and NSAIDs may be used alone or together. If they haven't worked within three months, go back to your doctor and see about changing your prescription.

SURGERY

Sometimes heavy bleeding can be cured by a minor operation called dilation and curettage (D&C), in which part of the womb lining is scraped out.

If you don't want to have any more children, surgeons can also use various methods to end the problem by removing the womb lining. If all else fails, a hysterectomy will put a stop to the bleeding for good. But this should be seen as a last resort.

I could have sung with the basses

'It started with horrendous periods in my thirties,' says Chris, a pharmacy assistant. 'I was on medication to control these for about seven years before having a hysterectomy. I later discovered that it was a male hormone I was given — I sang in a choir at the time and could have easily sung with the basses.

'The thing is, I was just given repeat prescriptions, the doctor saying it might be better by the time I got a hospital appointment, but of course it never was. Anyway, my doctor died and I had a new one who told me the maximum time I was meant to take this medication is two years. So I think it's important to research what you are given, as you may not be told the right information.'

Looking at the long term

Vasomotor symptoms may return when you stop taking the drugs that controlled them. The body then takes a while to adapt, as it does after menopause without drugs. In either case, the flushes and sweats wear off in time.

Urogenital symptoms stem from a lack of oestrogen, not from hormonal fluctuations, so they may continue in the long term. However, any treatment that helps for a while will delay deterioration over the long term. As the body adapts to less oestrogen, self-help techniques and over-the-counter remedies are usually enough to prevent discomfort.

Menopausal mood swings tend to wear off by themselves. Depression responds well to self-help therapies (see Chapter 4 on mind and mood). On average, researchers have found that women are happier after menopause than in their forties, and are often happier than in earlier life.

Professional help for depression

Sometimes the stresses and hormonal upheaval of menopause get too much to cope with alone. (Chapter 4 on mind and mood offers proven self-help measures.)

The best treatment a doctor can prescribe is probably a short form of psychotherapy. Two versions that have proved helpful with depression are cognitive behaviour therapy and problem-solving therapy. Both are offered as short courses of about 16 weeks – on the NHS, if you're lucky.

There may be a long waiting list for psychotherapy on the NHS. But you can also access it without going to your GP if you're prepared to pay. See 'Taking it further' for reputable organizations that can put you in touch with a trained practitioner.

If you're having severe enough mental health problems to be referred to a specialist, you may be offered longer forms of therapy. But it is quite unusual now for doctors to recommend this, as there is very little evidence to suggest it does much good for everyday problems such as depression.

Long-term processes such as psychoanalysis have not proved their value in any practical way. Indeed, some studies show that raking over the past can make you feel worse than ever – and not just in a short burst of 'healing pain' but in the long term too. The danger with any long-drawn-out form of psychotherapy is that you simply pore through all your past mistakes or grievances without learning how to move on.

Hypnotherapy has a bad track record for bringing up painful 'repressed memories' without healing the pain. Sometimes the supposed memory never happened: researchers have shown that it's quite easy to convince yourself of something that hasn't happened, and under hypnosis, people become even more convinced. Whether or not the 'repressed memory' turns out to be true, the treatment can easily do more harm than good. Bringing up a buried memory can be terrifying and destabilizing, and there's no guarantee that the therapist will then be able to help you cope with it.

On the other hand, many people have found hypnosis helpful for specific tasks focusing on the here and now, such as relaxation or coping with stressful situations. The danger seems to rest with anyone who seeks to take you back to an allegedly forgotten or suppressed trauma in your past.

IF YOU'RE FEELING DESPERATE

Your doctor may offer you antidepressants if things get really bad. When you've been depressed for a long time it can be hard to see a way out. Caught in a vicious circle, you haven't got the energy to do things that would lift your spirits. A short course of antidepressants may help to break the downward spiral and give you a breathing space in which to set up some healthy new habits such as taking exercise, getting outdoors more and spending time on activities (and people) that make you happy.

However, you shouldn't take antidepressants unless you really need them. The latest research shows that their benefits tend to be smaller than previously thought, and like any drugs they can have harmful side effects. Recently they've been linked with an increase in the rate of osteoporosis among users. Some research suggests that the selective serotonin-reuptake inhibitors (SSRIs), such as Prozac and many others, may occasionally trigger violent or suicidal actions.

On the other hand, antidepressants may be the best course of action for someone who is very seriously depressed. They may be what it takes to prevent suicide. It's a difficult path for a doctor to tread, and anyone taking these mood-altering drugs should be carefully monitored. If you are feeling desperate, make sure your doctor knows this and do follow the treatment that's prescribed.

If you do take antidepressants, you should follow the instructions to the letter, and don't come off them suddenly. Side effects may be unpleasant, and it may take time before you notice any good effects, but don't throw the tablets away if they don't seem to be having any effect. Even if they're not helping, they are changing levels of chemicals in your brain, and the effects of these drugs linger in the body for weeks. The greatest risk of suicide comes when people stop antidepressants suddenly, whether because of the side effects or because they think they'll cope better without drugs.

- ▶ *Considering suicide isn't the only danger sign. If you find yourself thinking about death, or of sleeping and not having to wake up, or just wishing you could find a way of escaping all your troubles, do seek immediate help.*
- ▶ *Never stop taking antidepressants suddenly, but wean yourself off them slowly under medical supervision.*
- ▶ *Never use antidepressants from one class, MAO inhibitors, within two weeks of taking SSRIs or SNRIs, which work in a different way. Even the herb St John's Wort should not be mixed with SSRIs or SNRIs. The combination can cause a fatal reaction.*

Do I need to take medicines as a preventive measure?

Every month, it seems, we hear about new drug discoveries that might save lives or prevent serious diseases. Sometimes the new drugs treat newly named conditions, such as pre-osteoporosis (a loss of bone density that could progress to osteoporosis), pre-diabetes or pre-hypertension. These are the conditions in which you're at high risk of developing a known serious health problem. But should they be treated as health conditions in themselves?

In recent years, drug success stories have been queried. Research sponsored by manufacturers has been found more likely to show their drug in a good light than independent research, and side effects are not always recorded. This casts doubt on the idea of taking a possibly harmful drug as a preventive measure, for a condition you might never have developed anyway. In January 2008, researchers reported that pre-osteoporosis drugs did little good for women with pre-osteoporosis, in comparison with the harmful side effects they could cause.

Researchers have found that lifestyle changes are more effective than drug treatment for all these pre-conditions. Medical experts advise people with pre-hypertension or pre-diabetes, for example, to eat more fresh produce, lose excess weight, cut down on unhealthy habits and take regular exercise. Healthy eating and exercise also help people with pre-osteoporosis protect their bones and build muscles to reduce the risk of falling.

COULD PREVENTIVE DRUGS BE CAUSING MY MENOPAUSAL SYMPTOMS?

▶ *Statin drugs, which reduce cholesterol levels and may reduce the risk of a heart attack, are being recommended to an ever-increasing number of healthy middle-aged people. Newer and stronger formulations in particular have been found to cause side effects including widespread muscle pain.*
▶ *Selective estrogen/oestrogen reuptake modulators (SERMs) such as raloxifene, prescribed to reduce the risk of fractures from osteoporosis, can cause hot flushes and night sweats.*

Summary

Various menopausal symptoms can be alleviated by treatments other than HRT. Several drugs may help to reduce hot flushes, though there is not a lot of evidence about their effectiveness or their side effects, especially in the long term. Heavy bleeding can be relieved by contraceptives, medicines, or by one of several possible operations on the womb. Your doctor may well recommend self-help measures such as dietary changes and exercise instead of medicines, or in addition to them.

Many 'pre-conditions' have now been identified as revealing that you are at increased risk of conditions such as diabetes, high blood pressure and osteoporosis. But there is no evidence that the drugs advertised as treating these pre-conditions work better than lifestyle changes. If your doctor thinks you are at high risk, even without symptoms, you may be offered preventive treatment. If you're not suffering and aren't at high risk, though, think hard before taking drugs aimed at preventing these conditions.

Action plan: selecting from twenty-first century options

1   *If you are concerned by any symptoms, such as heavy bleeding, see your doctor for a diagnosis. This should be done whether or not you wish to have treatment, as it may be caused by something other than the menopause. Prompt treatment could prevent it becoming more serious.*
2   *Ask your doctor about the different options available for your symptoms. Check about side effects, how big an improvement you're likely to see, how long it may take to show an effect, any restrictions that the treatment is likely to impose (for example, having to take drugs at a certain time of day or with food) and any long-term effects.*
3   *Ask about any lifestyle changes that could help. Get detailed information and carry these out if at all possible.*
4   *Express any preferences you have about hormones, other drugs, operations and lifestyle changes. This will help your doctor come up with a plan you will be motivated to follow.*
5   *If you start a course of treatment, follow the instructions exactly and take only the stated dose. Give it long enough to work – unless it causes serious side effects, in which case return to the doctor as quickly as possible and stop the treatment unless it is dangerous to do so (as with antidepressants).*

10 THINGS TO REMEMBER

1 *Several other drugs may be prescribed for women who want to take something for their symptoms but can't, or don't want to, use HRT.*

2 *Heavy bleeding could be relieved by the contraceptive Pill, non-steroidal anti-inflammatory drugs (NSAIDs), the blood-clotting drug tranexamic acid, or the contraceptive intrauterine system (IUS), which contains progestogen.*

3 *If other measures don't stem the flow, you may be offered an operation to stop heavy bleeding.*

4 *For hot flushes and night sweats, you may be offered tibolone, a drug that's intended to provide the same benefits as HRT, but which also increases cancer risks.*

5 *You may also be offered clonidine (usually prescribed to control migraines and high blood pressure), the epilepsy drug gabapentin or certain antidepressants.*

6 *Gabapentin's side effects include dizziness, tremor, clumsiness, fatigue and weight gain. Clonidine may cause nausea, drowsiness and dizziness.*

7 *Mood swings or depression may be treated with antidepressants.*

8 *Antidepressants often cause side effects similar to menopausal symptoms, such as disrupted sleep, confusion, loss of libido and weight gain. They may also cause dangerous emotional disturbances, especially if you stop taking them abruptly.*

(Contd)

9 *Drugs are available for people considered at risk of a condition such as osteoporosis or diabetes, aimed at preventing these 'pre-conditions' progressing any further. There is little evidence in their favour.*

10 *Most doctors prefer to treat 'pre-conditions' by recommending lifestyle changes, which are proven effective and have no side effects.*

10

Complementary approaches

In this chapter you will learn:
- *why there is little published evidence about complementary remedies*
- *what makes 'natural progesterone' natural*
- *how to use complementary therapies safely.*

The menopause, for most women, isn't a big enough deal to justify medical treatment. But women may well wish to reduce some inconvenient symptoms or give themselves a little more energy. That's why many women browse the complementary remedies shelf in pharmacies and supermarkets.

Taking a complementary approach to the menopause doesn't mean refusing to consider any medical help, whether needed or not. Nor does it mean putting your faith in untested products or bizarre treatments. It's just a question of looking at problems, and their solutions, from all angles.

Finding the evidence

This book aims to provide accurate information on all the subjects it covers. In the area of complementary and alternative therapies, however, reliable independent research is hard to come by. One reason is that product trials are prohibitively expensive; small companies genuinely can't afford to do them. The trials that have been done are generally undersized, and sometimes not well enough set up to meet the stringent standards of scientific publications.

Another reason is that no one stands to make much profit from sales of herbs, some of which can even be grown at home. As governments put little money into research these days, most funding comes from drug companies, which have no interest in alternative remedies. (Drug companies do own some herbal products and food supplements, but these only provide a small fraction of their income.) Charities fund a lot of research, but most of them cover specific diseases, rather than things that may just make you feel better when you're having a bad menopause day.

Finally, even independent research – the most reliable there is – may give misleading results. A study that was widely reported in 2002 as showing that St John's Wort was ineffective had been testing it for major depression, which it isn't intended to treat. Even so, the herb worked as well as the antidepressant drug sertraline, with which it was compared. And the placebo effect worked better than either, possibly suggesting that psychological therapies would be more useful. Sometimes the misleading reports stem from the researchers' or manufacturer's press release, which may put a spin on the study conclusions and may then be reported by a journalist who doesn't understand the science.

TRIED AND TESTED

The huge field of complementary and alternative therapies includes some wild extremes and fantastic beliefs. These aren't covered in this book, not only because there is no published evidence in their favour but – more importantly – because there is no convincing reason why they might be worth using.

Be cautious of any practitioner using non-standard devices, for example, claiming to diagnose allergies or 'imbalances' through measuring electric currents in your skin. Be especially cautious if these reveal conditions for which the practitioner sells a cure. If you decide to try an alternative remedy, please check first that it can't do any harm. Herbal remedies, for example, have caused many cases of liver damage (some fatal) when not prepared by experts.

However, the field also covers a lot of reasonable ideas and sensible approaches to health. It includes some ancient therapies that might have died out if they had never done any good – although the competence of people practising them today should always be investigated. And it is worth noting the studies that have been made of them, even if they don't meet all the tightest criteria. On top of that, people have very different reactions to remedies, whether pharmaceutical or complementary. That's why one person will get a drug side effect and another won't. This is especially true where hormones are concerned. So some women will benefit from taking common traditional remedies that haven't yet been proved effective. The most important point is to avoid anything that has not been proved safe.

Scientific researchers and publications pride themselves on their impartiality, but they can't always prevent a dislike of what seems 'unscientific' colouring their judgement. And many researchers could not continue working without support from drug companies, whose profits are reduced by alternative treatments and self-help therapies.

Some herbs and products have proved their worth, and their safety, over the years, even if they have never been put through scientific tests that would bring them official validation. Others have some published evidence for and against them, which we'll look at here.

HEALTHY CAUTION

As with any product that's meant to affect your health, the best course of action is to find out all you can, from reputable independent sources, about anything you're planning to use. Many remedies, such as exercises and certain foods, can be tried out for a few weeks. If they don't suit you or you don't think they're worth the effort, you can stop and try something else. But herbal remedies work more like drugs, in that they can have powerful effects and side effects. More deaths are caused by herbal medicines than by all other forms of complementary therapy added together.

'Natural' doesn't necessarily mean 'harmless' – some of the world's most deadly poisons are made directly from plants. And where research is concerned, 'no evidence of harm' isn't as good as 'evidence of no harm'.

However, the harm done by complementary remedies is insignificant compared with the thousands of adverse effects and deaths caused every year by medical treatment, especially drugs. This doesn't deny the value of orthodox medicines, or the fact that they may be used by people who are more seriously ill, but it does put concerns about herbal remedies into perspective. Be wary of anything that could harm you.

- ▶ *There's very little safety or quality control over products bought via the Internet. They may not even be what they're claimed to be. They can include ingredients not allowed in your own country.*
- ▶ *The same goes for individual blends made up for you by a herbalist, unless you know the practitioner is a member of a reputable organization and follows its code of practice.*
- ▶ *Anything that's legally sold in shops should be covered by stringent laws governing its safety and the claims manufacturers are allowed to make for it. This holds true in the English-speaking countries and the European Union. If a product comes under suspicion, it is normally removed from the shelves at once.*
- ▶ *Bear in mind, though, that a product might react with something else you're taking, or affect a health condition that may not have been diagnosed, or simply disagree with you. If it's strong enough to have good effects, it could have bad effects too.*
- ▶ *Because we still have much to learn about the way nutrients work together in their natural state and in our bodies, taking any kind of supplement or herbal remedy could cause an imbalance in the body's finely tuned chemistry.*

What are phytoestrogens?

These oestrogen-like compounds are found in certain plants (more about food sources in Chapter 12 on nutrition). Because they are weaker than our own natural oestrogen, or than HRT, they are thought to relieve menopausal symptoms without the health risks of HRT. There is a possibility, too, that they may protect against xenoestrogens – industrial pollutants that trick their way into the body by mimicking oestrogen, causing cancers and hormonal damage.

But there is some concern that the most powerful phytoestrogens might cause some of oestrogen's downsides too. Some studies suggest that taking phytoestrogen supplements for five years may cause thickening of the endometrium (womb lining), which can lead on to endometrial cancer. This is not yet certain.

Herbs on trial

Few of the following remedies have solid enough evidence behind them to convince orthodox health bodies that they can relieve the vasomotor symptoms. But smaller studies have suggested that some at least may reduce their frequency and severity. And others have been found to relieve different menopausal symptoms:

▶ **Black cohosh** (Actaea racemosa, Cimicifuga racemosa) *is believed by many to reduce hot flushes, although studies have had mixed results. It may cause stomach upsets or rashes in the short term, and is known to have caused liver damage in some cases. It may also reduce the effects of cancer drugs.*

- **Chasteberry** (Vitus agnus castus) *has been found to affect hormones including progesterone, and there is a little evidence that it may relieve breast pain.*
- **Devil's claw** (Harpagophytum procumbens) *was found a few years ago to be as effective against lower-back pain as the then standard painkiller rofecoxib. Rofecoxib has since been withdrawn from the market because of adverse effects on the heart, whereas devil's claw has shown no ill effects.*
- **Dong quai** (Angelica sinensis) *is a Chinese traditional remedy that has become popular in the past few years, but it hasn't been proved to reduce hot flushes. It may react with blood-thinning drugs and cause over-sensitivity to light.*
- **Evening primrose** (Oenothera biennis) *oil is widely used to relieve breast pain and swelling. Some women also find it helpful against hot flushes and mood swings, despite studies that found no effect.*
- ***Ginkgo biloba** has been found to improve blood circulation. Therefore it may (though there is less evidence for this) aid brain function, including memory.*
- **Ginseng** (Panax ginseng *or* Panax quinquefolius) *has been found to relieve mood swings, boost energy levels and improve sleep patterns. In some cases it may cause postmenopausal bleeding and breast pain, and may interact with warfarin, phenelzine and alcohol.*
- **Kava** (Piper methysticum) *may relieve anxiety, but has a number of serious side effects including liver disease. For this reason, it is not legally available in the UK.*
- **Linseed** (*flax seeds*, Linum usitatissimum) *have been found in some studies to reduce hot flushes, vaginal dryness and mood swings. They tackle menopausal symptoms from two angles, as they contain both omega-3 oils and phytoestrogen. The seeds work better than the oil, so grind up a couple of teaspoonfuls and swallow with plenty of water.*
- **Red clover** (Trifolium pratense), *a source of phytoestrogens, has a little evidence showing it may reduce hot flushes. A small three-year trial was reported in 2008 as showing that, unlike HRT, red clover did not increase the risk of tumours among*

*women who had a family history of breast cancer. In reality,
the study only looked at changes that might or might not lead
to future cancers. Red clover may react with blood-thinning
and cancer drugs.*

▶ **Sage** (salvia officinalis) *tea is a traditional remedy for
menopausal symptoms including hot flushes, but should not
be used if you have had breast cancer.*

▶ **St John's Wort** (Hypericum perforatum) *has been found
in many trials to reduce mild or moderate depression as
effectively as antidepressants, with fewer side effects. It has also
proved beneficial specifically for women in the perimenopause.
It should not be used in conjunction with antidepressants, and
it also reacts with many other drugs, including contraceptives
and asthma medication.*

Top tip

It is especially important not to take St John's Wort within
two weeks of taking an SSRI antidepressant, as this can
cause a fatal reaction. Black cohosh, red clover and sage may
reduce the effects of the breast cancer drug tamoxifen.

CHINESE HERBALISM

Chinese traditional medicine is usually made up to individual
prescriptions that may contain a dozen or more herbs. It's a holistic
discipline, covering many aspects of a patient's life and health as
well as the symptoms for which treatment is sought, in a effort to
put the entire system right. For this reason, it's hard to test how
well it works for menopausal problems.

If you try Chinese medicine, remember that it isn't a gentle
remedy like camomile tea. The prescriptions can be as powerful as
Western drugs. Some manufactured products have been tested in
laboratories and found to contain substances that should only be
available on prescription.

▶ *Ensure you're seeing someone qualified – although it's hard to
know if a certificate is for a genuine qualification.*

- *Don't persevere if you have any side effects.*
- *Don't use Chinese medicine if you're taking other drugs – they can interact badly.*

Insight

Some Chinese products on sale have been found to contain banned substances or high doses of drugs.

NATURAL PROGESTERONE

A product called 'natural progesterone' is also available in various forms. Though manufactured from the wild yam, it is made to be identical to the human hormone. It may be prescribed as a vaginal gel, or bought privately.

Insight

Surprisingly, natural progestogen has been found to be less effective than the more commonly used synthetic progestogen, which is not identical to the human hormone.

Wild yam (*Dioscorea villosa*) creams are also widely sold – not prescribed – as containing natural progesterone, or the hormone precursor DHEA. Although compounds in the plant can be converted to progesterone in a laboratory, the human body cannot process it in the same way. So the cream does not provide either progesterone or DHEA.

If you are taking an oestrogen-only form of HRT, do not use natural progesterone instead of a progestogen. It is not strong enough to counteract the risk of womb cancer from the oestrogen.

Should I be taking supplements?

Although dieticians stress the value of various nutrients in food, it's a mistake to take them out of context. It's very easy to cause a chemical imbalance in the body. Most women who are still menstruating need more iron in their diet, for example, especially if they're having heavy periods. But constipation is a common side effect of taking iron supplements. And if you're taking too much, they can cause serious damage to your heart and liver.

Vitamin E supplements are widely believed to reduce hot flushes, although there is little evidence to support this. However, taken in the long term they have been linked with serious harm including heart failure. Vitamin B6 has been found to reduce breast pain. But you could do more harm than good by taking a supplement that didn't include all the B vitamins, as they need to work together. Magnesium has been claimed to relieve hot flushes, though this has not yet been backed by evidence. But taking very little more than the recommended daily intake of one mineral can cause a deficiency of another.

Some large organizations specializing in women's health needs will recommend (and sell) combinations of supplements tailored to the individual. This might be a safe place to start if you wish to take supplements. See the Taking it further section for suggestions.

Top tip

If you're taking a remedy or supplement and feel worse, don't take another one to counteract the effects. Stop taking the first remedy. If you still feel worse, see your doctor.

Other options

Acupuncture has proved one of the most effective complementary treatments for menopausal symptoms, including hot flushes, night sweats, period pains, backache and insomnia. The pain relief is thought to result from the needles triggering the release of natural painkilling chemicals in the body. The effect on vasomotor symptoms hasn't been explained.

The effects of acupuncture on hot flushes remain a mystery –
either studies were inaccurate or western science doesn't yet
understand how acupuncture works.

Massage can ease the muscle pains, fatigue and headaches of the
perimenopause. By promoting deep relaxation, it can also relieve
insomnia.

The benefits of breathing exercises

'The best thing I did was learning breathing exercises in my
yoga class,' says Trish, a retired office manager. 'I liked
the classes and found yoga very calming when I did some
practice at home. Calming and uplifting. I didn't make
time to do it as much as I'd have liked. But the breathing
exercises were marvellous. I practised whenever I felt
stressed or dizzy. It worked like magic. I'm sure it could
stop a hot flush. The more I did it the better it was, maybe
because I became more confident with it. I'd recommend it
to anyone. Just simple breathing exercises.'

Self-help remedies

One technique that has been proved to control a range of
menopausal symptoms is meditation. It does more than just relieve
mood fluctuations. It has even been shown to reduce the frequency
and duration of hot flushes. It is also one of the most calming ways
of bringing your brain into focus, alleviating the rather frightening
cognitive symptoms such as forgetfulness and confusion. It's
neither a gift nor an achievement beyond most people's capability.
It works, and you can learn how to do it.

Breathing exercises work like a form of instant meditation. Research shows that practising for 15 minutes twice a day every day can halve the number of hot flushes you suffer, and reduce their intensity. Practising when you feel a hot flush starting may prevent it taking hold.

A simple meditation

Sitting with your back straight assists the meditative process – if you get backache, use a straight-backed chair for support. Apart from this, the only important thing to consider about position is to choose one in which you will be comfortable for your entire meditation period.

Close your eyes. If you've been hurrying, let your breath slow down to a natural pace. Then start counting your breaths. In-out, one. In-out, two. In-out, three. Up to ten, then start again. Keep your attention on your breathing: how the air feels as it enters and leaves your body, steadily counting.

The point is to focus fully on what you're doing and not to think about anything else. This allows your brain to switch into producing Alpha waves, a state in which things become smooth and effortless. If thoughts float into your mind, don't give them any attention. Just let them float out again.

When you've got the hang of it, you can focus on walking or carrying out any simple activity such as cleaning. It's all about focusing purely on what you're doing, without any active thoughts to prevent your brain switching to Alpha.

▶ *Do the same thing at the same time and in the same place every day.*
▶ *Set an alarm for ten minutes, so you don't get distracted by wondering how long you've been meditating.*

- ▸ *When you realize your mind has wandered, don't worry or criticize yourself. Just bring your attention back to the movement of breath and the count.*
- ▸ *Try to work up to 20 minutes or half an hour if you feel this is a realistic goal. However, bear in mind that it's much better to do a regular daily ten-minute meditation than to put it off till you've got half an hour free.*

Top tip

If you keep getting distracting thoughts when meditating, visualize wrapping them in a bubble and letting them drift away.

Insight

There are numerous forms of meditation, any of which can help to reduce stress and improve sleep patterns. Some people are more motivated to persevere if they've paid for a course. But it's possible to learn an effective technique from a book or in a simple lesson.

Breathing out anxiety

Breathing exercises can help to control stress and have been known to stop a hot flush before it gets properly started.

Put one hand on your chest and the other on your navel: if the lower hand doesn't move, you're not breathing deeply enough. Hasty, shallow breathing produces the stress hormone adrenaline. But a deep breath puts masses of oxygen into the bloodstream for an instant health boost to the whole body. No wonder it clears our heads: the oxygen is feeding our brain.

You'll get most benefit from this exercise if you're sitting with your back straight somewhere quiet, but it will work anywhere. If you're breathing fast, give yourself a minute to let it slow down naturally.

Then put your hands side by side on your abdomen, fingertips meeting at or just below the navel.

Take a deep breath in through your nose and feel the oxygen pouring into every corner of your lungs. Feel the abdomen rise and watch the movement parting your fingertips. Breathe out and do it again, this time feeling your chest expand slightly as well. Don't worry if it's not happening. If you're very used to holding your stomach in, you may need to push it out deliberately. The very act of making space there will let more air in.

▶ *After a few breaths, stop breathing deeply and let your natural rhythm establish itself, still breathing fully into the abdomen.*
▶ *You can have too much of a good thing, even oxygen. If you're feeling light-headed, either from breathing too deeply or from gulping in air under stress, breathe in and out of a paper bag a few times to restore the balance of oxygen and carbon dioxide.*
▶ *Check with your doctor before doing breathing exercises if you have epilepsy or high blood pressure.*

Summary

Many herbal remedies are marketed as relieving menopausal symptoms but few have been proved to help with the symptoms for which women most commonly seek relief – hot flushes and night sweats. Herbal remedies are more helpful in dealing with insomnia, headaches, fatigue and mind problems such as mood swings. Vitamin and mineral supplements are widely used but with little evidence in their favour. As it is easy to cause a nutritional imbalance by taking individual supplements, it would be better to seek professional help in tailoring a supplement regime – but bear in mind that most nutritionists do not have medically recognized qualifications. The safest course is to increase your intake through eating more nutrient-rich foods. A few other remedies have proved helpful, including acupuncture, massage and self-help techniques such as meditation.

Action plan: using remedies that are backed by evidence

1 *Learn and use one of the self-help mind-body techniques such as meditation, which have been proved to reduce many menopausal symptoms.*

2 *If you wish to try herbal remedies or food supplements, see what is available in pharmacies and health-food shops rather than on the Internet, as these are governed by safety regulations. Consider also taking nutritional advice from an organization or practitioner with medically recognized qualifications.*

3 *If you find a product you wish to try, follow the instructions exactly. Take it for at least six weeks to give it time to start working. But don't persevere if it is causing side effects.*

4 *If it doesn't make a significant difference and you wish to try something else, give up the first remedy rather than adding one on.*

10 THINGS TO REMEMBER

1 *Many complementary-therapy products, especially herbal remedies, are available to tackle menopausal symptoms.*

2 *Most of these have little evidence for their safety and effectiveness.*

3 *Taking single vitamins or minerals as supplements can cause harmful imbalances.*

4 *Some remedies have evidence in their favour. St John's Wort, for example, can relieve mild depression as effectively as an antidepressant. Acupuncture has proved effective in relieving some symptoms including period pain.*

5 *Anything strong enough to have a good effect may also have a bad one, so find out about side effects.*

6 *Herbal remedies cause many more adverse effects, including liver damage and deaths, than all other complementary therapies put together.*

7 *Herbal teas are usually harmless and may be backed by long use: chamomile, for example, aids sleep, peppermint can help digestion and sage may reduce hot flushes.*

8 *Products sold in UK shops have to meet European legal standards of quality.*

9 *There's no control over products bought on the Internet, either for safety or effectiveness.*

10 *Simple hands-on techniques are often the most effective. Massage, for example, has been proved to ease menopausal muscle pain and promote healthy sleep.*

11

A lifestyle that works for you

In this chapter you will learn:
- *what simple lifestyle changes could make this transition much easier*
- *why doctors may not recommend monthly breast examinations*
- *how to relieve many symptoms by improving your sleep quality.*

Many of the symptoms of the menopause can be alleviated with self-help measures, which cost nothing and have no harmful side effects. Healthy eating and fitness are two of the major self-help areas, and these are covered in other chapters in this book. Along with these, certain other do-it-yourself techniques can make a big difference to your chances of sailing through the menopause rather than feeling overwhelmed by it.

In this chapter, we'll look at those areas that have proved most valuable for physical symptoms of the menopause. Self-help for the psychological and emotional aspects is covered in Chapter 4 on mind and mood. Chapter 10 on complementary approaches gives details of other techniques that help during the menopause generally.

Almost anyone can benefit from making a few small changes, whether or not they're suffering from physical symptoms of hormonal change. As well as improving life now, they set you up for a healthier and more enjoyable life ahead.

One of your greatest needs during the menopause is good-quality sleep. Insomnia adds to many women's problems at this time. A number of different menopausal symptoms conspire to keep you awake: night sweats, restless legs, anxiety and muscle pain all rob you of the sleep that you now need more than ever. Learning the new habits that experts in the field call 'sleep hygiene' can put an end to insomnia and relieve the many other problems that it exacerbates.

This is also a good time to work on changing any bad habits that are now starting to take their toll. Smokers experience up to twice as many hot flushes as other women – that's as good a motive as any to give up a habit that, at this time of life, starts having a serious impact on your overall health. Excess weight, alcohol, a sedentary lifestyle and reliance on over-the-counter medicines can all whittle away at your health and vitality.

Insight

Lifestyle changes don't have to be hard work. One of the most valuable things you can do is to give yourself more time. Lying on the floor with a cushion under your knees to ease your back, sitting in meditation or allowing yourself time to digest your meal instead of rushing on to the next chore – all these help to relieve menopausal symptoms.

TREAT WITH RESPECT

A few lifestyle changes can prevent all kinds of niggling health conditions taking hold. Almost as importantly, you can avoid stepping onto the medicine treadmill.

Drugs are available for many of the minor problems that we all face at some time. But though they work faster than, say, taking exercise or learning to meditate, they don't necessarily work any better in the long term. And they can create all kinds of side effects. Once you start on one medicine, you may soon find yourself suffering a whole set of new symptoms. You could then be prescribed another drug for a problem you didn't realize was itself a drug side effect. And the second set of side effects could necessitate another medicine, which clashes with the first one.

Doctors are extremely pressed for time; they rarely have enough time to pore through your entire medical history, let alone work out the details of your individual health needs. You may not have a doctor's specialized knowledge, but you owe it to yourself to take the time required to work out what your body needs right now.

Some serious health conditions can only be treated with drugs. Obviously you need to take your doctor's advice if you are ill, or are at high risk – and the earlier the better. But drug treatment for minor conditions can end up making you worse than if you'd done nothing. A healthier alternative is to try all relevant self-help measures first. You don't need to take herbal remedies or supplements – they require specialist knowledge and may cause side effects of their own. Just try some lifestyle adaptations that are conducive to good health and an easy transition through the menopause.

Top tip
As lifestyle changes don't clash with other remedies – medical or complementary – you can always use them together.

Insomnia or unrefreshing sleep

Nothing short of disease saps our strength and vitality faster than insomnia or constantly broken sleep. Yet surveys suggest that one in three people feel they don't sleep enough.

Insight
Women suffer more from insomnia than men at any time of life, partly for hormonal reasons; PMS, for example, is linked with shallow sleep at that time of the month.

During the menopause we need a good night's rest more than ever. And this is the very time when many women find they can't get off to sleep, or are disturbed by the slightest sound, or wake up drenched in sweat. This not only leaves you needing more hours of sleep, it also disrupts the stages of sleep that you need to progress through each night.

Sleep doesn't just give us a chance to rest; it's also the time when we grow and when our bodies can repair any damage done during the day. Hormones play an important role: during the day we produce the adrenaline, noradrenaline and cortisol that keep us active but also contribute to wearing out our bodies. At night the production of those busy hormones drops off and we produce others, including growth hormone, to repair and rebuild.

This process can be disrupted by the hormonal changes of the menopause, as well as by late nights, shift work or even stress. We then produce too much of the daytime hormones, and not enough of those we need to replenish our health and energy.

A normal night starts with Stage 1, when you feel drowsy and may even have fragments of dreams despite not being really asleep yet. Then you slip away into Stage 2 – the longest part, taking up about half your sleeping time – then deep into Stages 3 and 4, when the brain waves slow down, the body does most of its repair work and you're hard to wake up. Next comes rapid-eye movement (REM) sleep, in which you're dreaming. Your muscles lose strength, to prevent you acting out your dreams or falling out of the window. (If you wake suddenly from REM sleep you may feel, terrifyingly, paralysed for a few moments before your body adjusts.) Then the cycle starts again.

It's now known that you need the right amount of each stage of sleep, and in the right order, to get the most from your sleep. You may feel constant fatigue despite thinking you've slept through the night. But if you were sleeping shallowly or being half-woken by heat or leg cramps, you may not have slept effectively.

Poor sleep exacerbates menopausal symptoms and may even be the main reason for some of them.

▶ *Your blood levels of the hormone cortisol are raised, making you feel stressed.*

▶ *Just one night's broken sleep dulls your brain functions, including your memory, alertness, attention span and ability to plan.*

▶ *The area of the brain most involved with sleep is the frontal area of the cerebral cortex, which is also responsible for speech, short-term memory and flexible thinking. This explains why we're so fuzzy and slow-witted after a bad night.*

▶ *Physically too, you feel the need of the healing and repairing hormones that are only released during sound sleep. Without it, your limbs may ache and everything is more effort.*

▶ *A poor sleeping pattern may even make you gain weight, unhealthily, in the form of fat. Poor sleep reduces your levels of growth hormone, which helps the body use food to build muscle rather than laying it down as fat, and which is produced during deep sleep. Lack of sleep can also make you feel hungrier during the day, as your body desperately seeks another source of energy.*

How can you tell if you're sleep-deprived? Sleep experts agree that few people genuinely thrive on much less than seven hours sleep a night. If you feel fatigued and irritable during the day, don't accept it as part of the menopause: you should be able to repair your broken patterns with the advice below.

What if you sleep like a log, but still wake up feeling groggy? Check whether it's something you've taken. Many drugs can leave you feeling thick-headed when you wake up – not only sleeping tablets but other common medicines such as codeine and antihistamines.

Depression is another common reason for feeling slow and heavy when you wake. It may wake you up before dawn, or it can cause poor sleep and frequent waking, which you may not remember in the morning.

Or you may simply not be sleeping anywhere near as well as you think. Some people have undiagnosed sleep disorders such as apnoea, in which breathing keeps being briefly interrupted. Such disorders become apparent at around this time of life. Snoring or waking with a headache are clues to this, but it really needs to be diagnosed and treated by a specialist.

HOW TO SLEEP BETTER

If you have trouble sleeping, a few simple changes should make a difference.

▶ *Get into a general habit of going to bed and getting up at the same time every day, whether you've slept well or not. But if you're really not ready for sleep, don't force yourself to go to bed until you do feel sleepy. Then get up at the normal time anyway – you should sleep better the next night.*

▶ *Take some exercise every day, or your body will still be restless when your brain is ready to sleep. If evening exercise wakes you up, try to fit it into your lunch hour.*

▶ *In the evening, don't watch action films, have arguments or do anything else that stimulates rather than helps you wind down.*

▶ *Don't eat a heavy meal late at night. Have dinner early, then have a hot drink (unless this wakes you up to go to the loo) and a light snack before bed.*

▶ *Create a calming bedtime routine – for example bath, peaceful music, prepare clothes for the next day – and follow it every night.*

▶ *An overheated bedroom can cause restless sleep. Leave a window open or, if you keep the heating on overnight, experiment by turning the thermostat down. For the same reason, have your bath warm rather than hot.*

> ▶ *If you're awake for more than 15 minutes, get up and go into*
> *another room. Read a book or do something useful so you*
> *don't fret about the time you're wasting.*

Top tip

If you have any night-time symptoms, set a 6 p.m. curfew on
eating spicy food, drinking alcohol or coffee and smoking.
Caffeine and nicotine can keep you awake. Alcohol causes
shallow sleep and can interfere with your breathing. Spicy
food and exercise can make you too hot.

Restless legs

Some people get an unpleasant, jumpy feeling in their legs that
stops them relaxing, and may even make their legs jerk noticeably.
Known as 'restless legs', this is something that tends to strike
women around the time of the menopause. It comes on most at
night, when it's not only uncomfortable but can wake you up and
stop you getting back to sleep.

Restless legs may be a symptom of illnesses, or possibly of a
mineral deficiency such as anaemia, which is often caused by heavy
periods. If your doctor finds that you're anaemic, you may be
prescribed iron supplements – don't take them otherwise, as they
do more harm than good if not needed. Just increase your intake
of healthy foods containing iron, magnesium, potassium and
calcium; see Chapter 12 on nutrition. Restless legs can also be
a side effect of drugs used to treat depression, anxiety, high blood
pressure, nausea or allergies. But it often strikes for no apparent
reason.

Staying fit, especially with yoga and other stretching exercises,
can reduce the likelihood of an attack. Keep a diary to work out
your individual triggers: many people find it's set off by anything
stimulating in the evening such as coffee, alcohol, cigarettes or
aerobic exercise.

When it happens, try massaging or stretching your legs, or if you can't settle down, go for a walk. You could also experiment with baths and compresses: some people find warmth helps while others prefer cold.

Night sweats

These are the nocturnal version of hot flushes, so all the same advice applies. They are more of a nuisance in that they happen when you're trying to sleep, and may even be severe enough to wake you up. Some women sweat so profusely that they have to change the sheets before they can get back to sleep. On the other hand, being at home allows you to take measures, such as standing naked in front of an electric fan, that aren't recommended in the workplace.

In a vicious circle, night sweats can both cause insomnia and be exacerbated by it. Taking the advice given in this chapter to improve your sleep patterns could reduce your incidence of night sweats too.

▶ *Stock up on pure cotton sheets and pillowcases. Synthetics and cotton-synthetic mixes may be non-iron, but they trap the heat. And who says you have to iron sheets anyway?*

▶ *If you have a partner who feels the cold, consider using a single quilt each; yours can be swapped for a lighter weight one or a sheet when necessary.*

▶ *Wear a cotton nightdress, and keep others ready to change into. This may save having to change the sheets in the middle of the night.*

▶ *Reduce the thermostat in the bedroom, or keep a window open. Preferably, turn heating off overnight.*

▶ *Wise manufacturers have realized there's a market for 'cooling pillows', nightwear in special fabrics that wick moisture away, and even a high-tech mattress that regulates the temperature! Find them online.*

Body lotion heat

'I get an awful lot hotter if I'm smothered in body lotion after the bath than if I'm not,' says Sue. 'I've had some really bad night sweats with body lotion on. I'm convinced it does make you hotter – it's a physical barrier.'

Hot flushes

That sudden rush of heat to the head and chest is the menopausal bugbear that's most likely to send women to their doctors. The following suggestions have all proved to help.

▶ *When you feel a flush starting, do some breathing exercises or meditation. See Chapter 10 on complementary approaches.*

▶ *Run cold water over a pulse point – the quickest way to cool down, as your blood is close beneath the skin there. Your wrists are easiest to reach, or you can press something cold against the pulse in the side of your throat.*

▶ *Lose excess weight – this is one of the main triggers for hot flushes that you can control.*

▶ *Stop smoking – this could halve the number of hot flushes you suffer.*

▶ *Cut down on caffeine, alcohol and spicy foods.*

▶ *Dress in light cotton layers that are easy to take off.*

▶ *Carry a fan, and have one on your desk at work. You can even keep a miniature battery-operated fan in your handbag.*

▶ *Be an inventive shopper. Pharmacies and department stores sell all kinds of devices that can help you cool down. Some specially made products can be tracked down online with a search for 'cooling products'. Otherwise, a couple of gel packs, intended for sports injuries, can be kept in the freezer and one*

taken out with you every day. Freezable sleeves to cool wine
bottles can be used the same way, and the champagne size can
even be slipped over your wrist. Don't overdo it, though – you
don't want to get frostbite.

However, the most creative way of coping with sudden changes
of inner temperature is to change the way you feel about them.
A hot flush isn't harmful in itself, and some women find it
relieves a build-up of tension. For many women, it's only even
a nuisance because they feel embarrassed and flustered by this
visible sign of hormonal activity. You can decide to think of it
instead like a valve mechanism, protecting you by letting out
excess heat; looking at it this way neutralizes the emotional
content, which is what causes most of the distress. Some women
even say they feel invigorated by a hot flush – or what they call
a 'power surge'.

Top tip
If hot flushes are really bothering you, keep a self-help kit
handy: a fan, a rosewater spray, a light jacket or cardigan
(anything that can be slipped off rather than pulled over your
head), and cooling packs ready in the freezer.

Plumbing improved but thermostat haywire

'As soon as gynaecological plumbing ceases its monthly
inconvenience, you find your internal climate-control
thermostat goes haywire,' sighs Judith, who works for an
environmental organization. 'For me, hot flushes and night
sweats were a problem for about two years. The night-
time overheating and lying awake was the most annoying
symptom. Trickiest to cope with? Flushes coming on while
in work meetings.

(Contd)

'I found one way to cope was to acquire a stock of elegant fans to keep in your handbag and flutter when you feel tropical. These are especially useful if you travel by London Underground during summer, when all passengers share a good approximation of the hot flush experience.

'Second, build up your collection of cardigans and little jackets that can be unobtrusively unbuttoned and slipped off, rather than jumpers that demand to be pulled over your head. Particularly, give up rollneck tops for the duration. Third, relax.'

Dryness

Skin and hair may dry out surprisingly quickly around this time. Some women think they've developed eczema when their skin becomes flaky. In reality, they may just need to start buying hand cream, give up harsh hair products or open a window instead of switching on the air-conditioning.

This is a good time to review your make-up and hair-care routine, and to experiment with different moisturizers and shampoos. Fill a pump-action spray bottle with water to spritz your skin during the day; a dash of rose water makes it more soothing.

Many women find their eyes become uncomfortably dry at this time, and HRT doesn't help – in fact, it can make them worse. If you spend a lot of time at a computer, you probably don't blink enough unless you consciously remember to do so.

Simple eye drops – 'artificial tears' – are the best relief; stronger ones contain chemicals that can cause irritation. Common-sense tactics such as avoiding air-conditioning and putting bowls of water near radiators can also help. Splash your face with cool water every now and then.

Vaginal dryness can lead to thrush and cystitis as well as making sex uncomfortable. See Chapter 7 on sexuality for information about the many lubricants and other soothing products available.

Breast care

Every woman over 50 is advised to have regular mammograms, as the risk of breast cancer increases with age. In the UK, you will be invited to have one every three years. If your invitation goes astray, go to your doctor and ask to be referred for a mammogram. In some countries, doctors recommend mammograms as often as once a year.

However, cancer experts in the UK no longer advise women to do a set breast examination every month, as this advice didn't prove to save lives. Instead, they say, we should just have a relaxed awareness of our breasts. Each woman should come to know what is normal for her, and keep an eye on any changes. You can take a moment to look at them while you're dressing, and feel them while you're relaxing in the bath.

If you're still having periods, for example, it may be normal for your breasts to feel lumpy and uncomfortable for a few days before your period starts. Even if you've had a hysterectomy, the same may happen each month when you would have had a period, until the time when they would have stopped naturally. When you've stopped having periods, your breasts are likely to be softer, without any lumpiness or other monthly changes.

You should be aware of what changes need to be reported to your doctor. Look out for:

▶ *any changes in the outline or shape of your breast, especially if revealed by arm movements or lifting your breast*

- *puckering or dimpling of the skin*
- *sharp pains, and any pain or discomfort in one breast, especially if it is new or persistent*
- *any lumpiness, thickening or 'orange-peel' skin on a breast or in an armpit*
- *nipple discharge, rash or bleeding, and any change to the feel or appearance of a nipple*
- *heat, redness or rash.*

If you're taking HRT you should be extra vigilant, and breast tenderness may be a valuable warning sign. Recent research suggests that women on HRT whose breasts become more tender are more likely than other HRT users to develop breast cancer.

Also, care for your breasts by making sure your bra is the right size. They need more support as we age, especially if they are large. According to manufacturers, most women wear the wrong size – and having got in the habit, they stick to it throughout their lives. We commonly choose a larger chest measurement and smaller cup size than we really need.

A trained fitter in a department store or specialist bra shop will find the size that fits perfectly. You may be surprised at how much younger it makes you look, too, providing an instant psychological boost.

A well-fitting bra protects your breasts (not from cancer, alas, but from other damage) and reduces the discomfort as hormones fluctuate. If your breasts change in size and shape during your menstrual cycle, it's worth being fitted for two or even three sizes of bra to suit all times of the month.

It has to be said that some people believe wearing a bra can harm breasts by impeding blood and lymph circulation. It's true that our distant ancestors managed without bras. But they were a lot thinner than we are, and their life expectancy was much lower.

Back care

Rare is the woman who reaches menopause without having ever suffered backache. The spine is a complicated structure, and hormonal changes weaken some of the muscles and ligaments holding it in place. Luckily, there are many things you can do both to relieve the pain and to prevent it coming back.

POSTURE

Most of us slouch. When we try to straighten up, we arch our lower backs, putting a strain on the spine.

- *Stand up, feet side by side and a little apart, weight evenly between your feet.*
- *Imagine lengthening your spine upwards.*
- *Raise your shoulders and drop them a few times.*
- *Try to feel your spine in a natural curve and all your body in a neutral position – nothing sagging or bent or unnaturally rigid.*

If you're not sure whether you've got it, experts such as those teaching the Alexander Technique or Feldenkrais can put you straight.

FURNITURE

Ensure you're working at the right height, whether at a desk, in your kitchen or just sitting down: you should be able to put your feet on the floor when sitting on a chair or sofa.

ACTIVITY

Modern life means most of us spend most of the time sitting down. Back-care specialists beg us to do the opposite. Walking instead of sitting in a car or bus, visiting a colleague rather than sending an email, even lying flat on the floor rather than slumping into an armchair – all of these are kinder to your back.

DEALING WITH PAIN

For sudden back pain, it's a long time since doctors recommended bed rest. That was proven in the 1990s to do more harm than good. Obviously, if it's a serious injury you'll need hospital treatment at once. But otherwise, you're no longer advised to lie down, to rest for as long as you need or to give it time to wear off by itself.

Try to keep on with all your normal activities, even if they cause some discomfort. Don't restrict your life. Once you start making room for the pain, it sets in, both physically and psychologically. Back specialists now recommend staying at work if you can, and not lying down unless you have to. If you keep up your normal activities you'll have less pain in the long term.

Also, doctors say, the sooner you fix a back problem, the better your chances of a complete cure. Letting it drag on is likely to compound the damage and lead you into bad postural habits that make the problem worse. If it hasn't cleared up in three or four days, doctors may recommend a visit to a massage therapist, physiotherapist, chiropractor or osteopath.

▶ *Don't bypass your GP, who should be able to make a diagnosis and check that the pain isn't caused by an undiagnosed condition.*
▶ *If you choose to see a practitioner, contact the governing body for each profession to find a list of members in your area. Personal recommendation is useful too.*
▶ *Never let anyone touch your spine unless they have recognized qualifications – anyone can set up an 'institute' and award diplomas and letters after their name.*
▶ *If your back pain drags on, ask your doctor if there's a local back-care clinic. Some hospitals run tailored programmes of exercises and weekly classes.*

Shopping list

A few useful items can make a big difference to your health and comfort during the menopause. It's worth doing the research, shopping around and investing some money to get exactly what you need:

▶ *good shoes to support not only your feet and legs but also your spine*
▶ *correctly fitted bras to protect your breasts and prevent premature ageing*
▶ *cooling products and devices*
▶ *cotton nightwear, bed linen and easy-to-layer clothes*
▶ *a firm mattress, and possibly a sofa that fits you*
▶ *anything that makes you feel good without getting you into debt!*

Top tip
Exercising three times a week doubles a smoker's chance of giving up smoking successfully, and halves her risk of putting on weight.

Creating new habits

When considering advice about health and lifestyle, you know best what suits you and what you're likely to stick with. But remember that people change over the years. Old habits don't necessarily die hard, if you're ready to drop them. Something you've always done may not suit you any more. Motivated by the wish to stay healthy and active, you may find you're ready to move on.

▶ *Stop smoking. Stubbing out your last cigarette is one of the biggest favours you can do for yourself at this time of life. The fact that smokers reach the menopause on average two years before non-smokers, and have twice as many hot flushes, underlines the amount of harm tobacco does to your hormones.*

▶ *Slow down. Hormonal effects on the brain and central nervous system can make you feel clumsy. The simplest way of preventing falls and accidents is to give yourself more time to do things. If necessary, accept that you're not going to get as much done. Constipation, which many women start to suffer at this time, can also be alleviated by just giving yourself more time; keep some magazines in the loo as encouragement.*

▶ *Be kind to your legs. The powerful beat of your heart sends blood surging around your body in the arteries. But the blood's journey back to your heart is harder work. The valves in your leg veins, which help to stop it slipping backwards, are weakened by menopausal changes. This causes varicose veins, which are not only unsightly but make your legs ache and discourage you from taking exercise. To reduce the risk, try to avoid sitting with your legs crossed, putting on weight and spending a lot of time standing still. Give them a welcome break by sitting or lying with your feet raised.*

▶ *Go for a walk every day, thinking of nothing except what you see around you. Give up perfectionism, don't brood on problems and stop worrying about things you can't control. In other words, prevent stress. Although you can't prevent all the situations that put pressure on you, you can change the way you experience them, making yourself effectively stress-resistant.*

Insight

If you're taking drugs, developing side effects and taking other drugs to deal with those, consult your doctor to see if you can come off any of them. You may need to wean yourself off some medicines rather than stopping suddenly. Lifestyle changes may help with the transition.

Summary

Certain lifestyle changes can markedly reduce any menopausal symptoms you suffer. A few have proved especially effective.

The ones detailed in this chapter are those most likely to have a useful effect on the most common symptoms. Improving your sleep patterns will also alleviate many problems, including some you may not have realized were sleep-related. Various other symptoms of the menopause can be relieved with minor adjustments to everyday life.

Action plan: using your lifestyle to enhance your life

1 *If any symptoms of the menopause are bothering you, make a commitment to yourself to take action to relieve them.*
2 *Draw up a schedule making time for all the lifestyle changes you want to put into practice. For example, allocate yourself ten minutes every morning for meditation, half an hour of exercise three to five times a week, at least two periods a week of downtime with friends and roughly the same amount of time for yourself alone.*
3 *The schedule will probably seem overcrowded. Look through the other things that take up your time and see what you could leave out. Make your health and wellbeing a priority.*
4 *Week by week, check that you're keeping up with the things you need to do. Make adjustments where necessary, but don't let your own needs slip to the bottom of the priority list.*

10 THINGS TO REMEMBER

1 *Simple changes can alleviate most perimenopausal symptoms, as well as improving your prospects for long-term health.*

2 *They cost little or nothing and can be tailored to suit your lifestyle and level of motivation.*

3 *Lifestyle changes don't generally clash with medical treatments, and may even improve their effects.*

4 *If you have insomnia or poor sleep patterns, your tiredness will exacerbate many other symptoms. So this is one of the first things to tackle.*

5 *Drawing up a list of intended changes and a timetable helps to fit them into your everyday life.*

6 *Don't sabotage yourself by trying to make too many changes at once, or setting unrealistic goals such as losing lots of weight.*

7 *Start by looking up the symptom that bothers you most and make the easiest-looking changes that are recommended. Quick improvements, even if small, will motivate you to continue.*

8 *Meditation and breathing exercises reduce the stress that accompanies hot flushes and can sometimes defuse a hot flush that's already starting.*

9 *Use resources that can help you make any large changes, such as government helplines for giving up smoking.*

10 *There are websites and online communities for almost any concern, which you can find through an online search for relevant words.*

12

Nutrition

In this chapter you will learn:
- *how foods can affect the hormones*
- *what combinations of foods can help relieve menopausal symptoms*
- *why there is a debate about soy foods.*

We are what we eat. So it's not surprising that food can cause or cure many of the everyday health conditions we encounter. What we eat affects hormones as much as any other part of our system, so the right choice of food can make a useful difference to menopausal symptoms. Iron-rich foods such as meat replace the iron lost through heavy bleeding, for example. A spicy curry, on the other hand, could trigger a violent hot flush.

> **Insight**
> Hot flushes can be triggered by hot foods, either high-temperature or super-spicy. So avoid food or drinks that nearly burn your tongue (which is unhealthy anyway). Swap chillies and fierce curries for milder alternatives. Cutting down on caffeine and alcohol could also reduce the frequency and severity of vasomotor symptoms.

The idea of a balanced diet has changed dramatically since little over a century ago, when vegetables were considered as worthless ballast, only good for easing hunger if you couldn't afford enough meat.

Vegetables and fruits are now known to be the most essential foods we eat, and any healthy diet should be based on the widest possible range of them. Again, research is coming up with new findings all the time. But nothing challenges that now well-established fact. The new findings simply reveal more and more benefits in ever finer detail: cruciferous vegetables, such as broccoli, for reducing the risk of ovarian cancer, for example, and grapes for helping to keep arteries clear.

The hormonal upheaval of the perimenopause puts your body under pressure. So you need the support of a healthy, easily digested diet that will strengthen your immune system, keep your mind clear and top up your energy levels. This healthy diet will help to even out hormonal fluctuations.

Then you can add foods to address particular symptoms that are troubling you. However, many women will find that simply eating a healthy, hormone-friendly diet is enough to reduce or even clear up the symptoms anyway.

Importantly, you should reduce the amount of processed food and sweet or fatty snacks you eat. Junk food not only takes the place of foods that could be enhancing your life, but has a lot of harmful effects too. Sweet snacks destabilize your blood-sugar levels, while saturated fat clogs up your arteries.

A healthy eating plan should see you comfortably through the menopause and into the years that follow in the best shape you've ever achieved.

CAN'T I GET ALL THIS FROM SUPPLEMENTS?

With more information coming out all the time about the complex roles of different natural chemicals inside each plant, it's become clear that taking supplements isn't an alternative to a healthy diet. A tablet containing a few isolated vitamins or minerals doesn't come near the range and finely tuned balance of nutrients you get when you bite into an apple or some stir-fried vegetables.

Some tablets can even be harmful – taking iron supplements, for example, can cause heart and liver disease. Even low-dose tablets could cause a dangerous vitamin or mineral imbalance. And it's easy to overdose on supplements. See Chapter 10 on complementary approaches for more information.

Insight
Supplements provide nutrients outside their natural context and in concentrated doses, throwing your body's levels out of balance.

Eating for a healthy change

This plan will provide all the nutrients you need to stay strong and reduce hormonal fluctuations as much as possible. It will also help you shed fat if you need to, and maintain a healthy weight. If you suffer from mood swings or fluctuating energy levels, it should even these out too.

Our food requirements change at different times of life, and this plan is intended for an average woman going through the perimenopause. However, it is based on the healthiest principles: the widest possible range of vegetables, and of fruit (in smaller amounts if your weight is an issue) and as little processed food as possible.

It takes account of the glycaemic index (GI), which rates foods by the speed at which the body turns them into sugar. Most of the foods in this plan are low- or medium-GI, which maintain steady blood-sugar levels. This in itself reduces the risk of diabetes and could be enough to smooth out mood swings.

Insight
The glycaemic index (GI) indicates how quickly a food releases sugar into the bloodstream. Low-GI options are the most wholesome and natural, and include most vegetables and wholemeal cereals. High-GI foods – often refined products such as white flour – raise blood-sugar levels very quickly, which can lead to mood swings and exhaustion.

You'll be eating to strengthen your body, while letting go of unnecessary fat. If you've slipped into the habit of eating processed foods, this could be the moment when you discover a whole new world of taste and freshness.

Check with your doctor before making any substantial change to your diet, especially if you have a known health condition. If you have special nutritional needs, these must take precedence. If you are doing a lot of heavy work, your requirements may be different again.

THE HEALTHY EATING PYRAMID

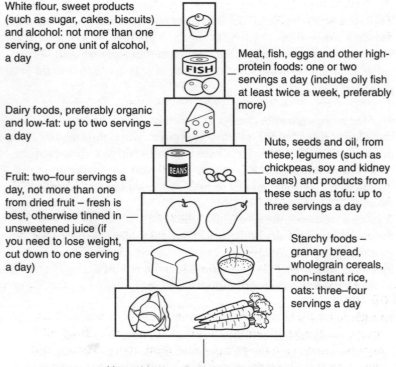

White flour, sweet products (such as sugar, cakes, biscuits) and alcohol: not more than one serving, or one unit of alcohol, a day

Meat, fish, eggs and other high-protein foods: one or two servings a day (include oily fish at least twice a week, preferably more)

Dairy foods, preferably organic and low-fat: up to two servings a day

Nuts, seeds and oil, from these; legumes (such as chickpeas, soy and kidney beans) and products from these such as tofu: up to three servings a day

Fruit: two–four servings a day, not more than one from dried fruit – fresh is best, otherwise tinned in unsweetened juice (if you need to lose weight, cut down to one serving a day)

Starchy foods – granary bread, wholegrain cereals, non-instant rice, oats: three–four servings a day

Vegetables – unlimited amounts, at least five servings a day and preferably more

The healthy eating pyramid.

This pyramid shows what proportion of different foods you should eat each day. The peak of the pyramid – sweets and alcohol – is the only layer that is unnecessary; it's fine to leave it out altogether if you wish.

RULES OF THUMB

One serving of most foods is roughly 80 g (3 oz). In general, this is about as much as you can hold in the palm of your hand. Use the following as a guide:

- *beans and pulses: 2 heaped tablespoonfuls*
- *berry-sized fruit: one small bowl of strawberries, grapes, etc.*
- *bread rolls: the size of your fist*
- *bread: one slice*
- *cheese: a 2.5 cm (1 inch) cube, about the size of the top joint of your thumb*
- *cooked fruit and vegetables: 2–3 tablespoonfuls*
- *dried fruit, nuts and seeds: about a handful*
- *fruit juice: a 150 ml glass*
- *fruit, large: one big slice of melon, etc.*
- *fruit, medium-sized: one apple, pear, etc.*
- *fruit, small: two plums, satsumas, etc.*
- *meat and fish: a piece as big and thick as the palm of your hand*
- *oils and fats: 1 teaspoonful*
- *pasta sauce: a ladleful as big as your fist*
- *pasta: a bundle of dry spaghetti 2.5 cm (1 inch) across, or two handfuls when cooked*
- *salad: one small mixed side salad.*

Top tip

Organic foods, produced with minimal use of chemicals and drugs, are the healthiest you can buy. If you can't afford all organic, choose the most important: meat, dairy produce and eggs, plus leafy vegetables and salads and anything grown out of season, as the non-organic versions of these are likely to have been heavily sprayed.

Changing needs

As you progress towards the menopause, your body's needs change to meet new challenges. So your best choice of foods may change over the next few years.

You may have heavy periods in the early stages of perimenopause, for example, which require a lot of iron. We're also advised to eat calcium-rich foods to keep bones strong, but calcium can reduce your body's ability to use iron. So when your periods are heavy you need to concentrate more on iron-rich food. Don't give up calcium-rich dairy foods, though, because they do so much good beyond protecting your bones.

As your periods become lighter, you no longer need so much iron, and in fact having too much iron becomes unhealthy. After your periods stop, you continue to need a good supply of calcium, and of protein to retain muscle strength. However, you're not recommended to eat a lot of meat after the menopause, because it can increase the risk of heart disease. Small servings of lean organic meat are the best compromise, along with protein from other sources, especially oily fish.

Low-fat dairy food is rich in calcium, and yogurt is especially easy to digest.

Nutrient sources

Essential nutrients are found in a wide range of foods, especially fresh fruit and vegetables. This list includes some particularly good sources of nutrients. But this is only the tip of the iceberg – try eating as many different fruits and vegetables as you can to cover some of the many other nutrients they contain.

▶ **carotenoids:** *main sources are red and orange-coloured fruits and vegetables; green leafy vegetables for beta carotene and lutein*

- ► **vitamin B6:** *spinach, peppers (capsicums), garlic, tuna, cauliflower, banana*
- ► **B vitamins generally:** *mushrooms, green leafy vegetables, asparagus*
- ► **vitamin C:** *many fruits, especially berries, kiwi fruit and citrus; green leafy vegetables, salad items, broccoli, brussels sprouts*
- ► **vitamin E:** *green leafy vegetables, sunflower seeds, almonds, olives, peppers, brussels sprouts, tomatoes, blueberries, broccoli*
- ► **vitamin K:** *green vegetables, carrots*
- ► **calcium:** *green leafy vegetables, dairy products, sesame seeds, green beans, garlic, tofu, kelp*
- ► **iodine:** *sea vegetables, dairy products, eggs, strawberries, fish*
- ► **iron:** *liver, beef, green leafy vegetables, lettuce, tofu, mustard greens, chick peas*
- ► **magnesium:** *spinach, courgettes, broccoli, seeds*
- ► **omega-3 fatty acids:** *salmon, flax seeds, walnuts, cauliflower, cabbage, tuna, soybeans, tofu, green leafy vegetables*
- ► **potassium:** *green leafy vegetables, mushrooms, brussels sprouts, broccoli, apricots, ginger, strawberries, avocado, banana*
- ► **protein:** *tuna and other oily fish, venison, liver, spinach, tofu, Portobello mushrooms, soybeans, cheese, eggs, beans, dairy products*
- ► **zinc:** *liver, beef, mushrooms, spinach, sea vegetables, green leafy vegetables, dairy produce, seeds.*

Symptomatic relief

The healthy eating plan in this chapter should go a long way towards relieving symptoms as well as improving your all-round health and vitality.

In addition, some women find certain foods helpful for individual symptoms. The suggestions below are not intended to replace a balanced diet. Foods that do you good when eaten in normal amounts can make you ill if you eat too much of them. And no matter how healthy an individual food is, it can't give you all the nutrients you require.

Try seeking out some of the foods that are rich in the suggested nutrients, and adding some to your everyday healthy diet.

Insight

On top of eating a healthy diet, you can tackle many symptoms by eating more of certain foods, such as potassium-rich fresh vegetables and salads to relieve fluid retention. Also, avoid ingredients that could trigger an attack, such as caffeine if you get restless legs.

DIGESTIVE PROBLEMS

The hormonal changes of the perimenopause have several effects on the way we digest and metabolize food. Because of the effects on various different organs, including the stomach and gall bladder, many women find they feel hungrier, are less easily satiated, suffer more indigestion and put on weight more easily, even if they don't eat more.

Peppermint, in any form, has been proven to relieve most kinds of indigestion, as it relaxes the muscles and helps to relieve the spasms which cause griping pains. But if you suffer from heartburn, peppermint may make it worse by weakening the valve that prevents acid rising into your oesophagus. When you're suffering from indigestion, sit upright and undo any tight clothing. If you're in bed, prop yourself up on pillows.

If you feel sick, have some ginger, again in any form, as it is an equally proven remedy. Both peppermint and ginger are easy to keep at hand in the form of herbal tea bags.

A drink of hot water can relieve a sharp abdominal pain if it's caused by wind. Or try massaging your abdomen with your fist, starting in the lower right-hand corner by your hip bone, up and across under your ribs, continuing in big clockwise circles.

Indigestion is exacerbated by smoking, alcohol, coffee and fatty foods; some people also find it is triggered by tomatoes or chocolate. You can reduce its recurrence by eating slowly and not having anything bigger than a snack late at night. Raw fruit and vegetables can cause indigestion in some people; rather than giving up those foods, try eating them cooked.

A healthy diet reduces the risk of constipation, as you're eating plenty of fresh fruit, vegetables or salad every day. But if your bowel moves slowly, try soaking a handful of dried fruit such as raisins in fruit juice and having this compote as an evening snack. If your bowel habit has changed suddenly, see your doctor, as this can be a sign of illness.

COGNITIVE FUNCTIONS

The first thing to do for your brain each day is to have breakfast. Researchers have found that people who have eaten a healthy breakfast do better in written and verbal tests than those who haven't eaten. You can think faster, reason more clearly and remember things better once you've given your brain some fuel to work with.

For the same reason, don't skip meals – the time you gain will be lost because you're not using it effectively. Low blood sugar can actually cause confusion and forgetfulness.

Nutrients that are especially useful to the brain include omega-3 oils, and the B group of vitamins.

HEADACHES AND MIGRAINE

Most migraine sufferers know that certain foods will trigger their shattering headaches, and ordinary headaches may also be caused this way. Coffee is an odd substance because, while some people find it triggers a migraine, others say that two strong cups at the start of an attack can ward it off.

Common trigger foods include chocolate, cheese and dairy produce, citrus fruits, alcohol, fried foods, nuts, meat, wheat, tomatoes, onions, corn, apples, bananas and the sweetener aspartame. Many sufferers are sensitive to tyramine, found in sour or fermented foods such as aged cheeses, pickled herrings, soy sauce and beer. Cut down on saturated fat, to improve circulation.

Ginger can ease the pain of headaches and migraine. Calcium-rich foods may also help, and magnesium has proved effective in treating or easing migraine and hormone-related headaches in several studies. If low blood sugar is a trigger, eat little and often.

HOT FLUSHES

Soy foods and sea vegetables are among the richest sources of the phytoestrogens that can work as a gentle, natural alternative to hormone replacement (see 'Do soy foods help or harm?' in this chapter). For women whose thyroid gland may be underactive or over-sensitive to soy, foods rich in iodine may counteract any ill effect. Foods rich in vitamin E are also helpful.

FLUID RETENTION

Foods high in salt encourage the body to retain fluid, exacerbating the puffy effects suffered by so many women at times during the perimenopause. Sugar may add to the problem. Processed foods are the main source of both for most women. Eating fresh fruit, vegetables and salad supplies potassium, which counteracts the unhealthy effects of too much salt.

Some people find that eating more fruit and vegetables makes their abdomen swell. But this is a different problem. It may take your digestive system a while to adjust to a sudden increase in your intake of fresh produce, but this is a natural diet and you should soon feel the benefits, first of all in curing constipation. If you have a sensitivity to fruit sugars, they may ferment in your intestine, meaning the swollen stomach is caused by wind, not fluid retention. The solution is to eat fruit in small amounts, leaving at least an hour between so you have time to digest it properly.

PAINFUL PERIODS

This can be caused by the hormonal fluctuations of perimenopause and can be eased by eating foods that balance the hormones. Eat a diet rich in essential fatty acids, especially fish oils. Cut down on fatty food and have plenty of fibre from fruit and vegetables, which may help to control hormone metabolism. Magnesium-rich foods may also help.

BREAST PAIN

Breast tenderness is often linked with fluid retention. Sufferers often find their abdomen swells uncomfortably before a period too. Get plenty of potassium by eating green vegetables or salad daily. Avoid salt, sugar, coffee, tea and soft drinks.

RESTLESS LEGS

Foods rich in iron, magnesium, calcium and potassium can help relieve the unpleasant feeling of jumpiness in your legs. Cut down on caffeine and alcohol, especially in the evening.

MUSCLE PAIN

Eat foods rich in unrefined carbohydrates, such as wholemeal bread, potatoes and fruit to increase the brain's production of the natural painkiller serotonin. Cut down on fatty foods, which may increase inflammation.

JOINT PAIN

Eat plenty of oily fish, since these are rich in the fatty acids that counteract inflammation. Fruit and vegetables provide vitamin C and other nutrients that help repair damaged joints, along with helpful carotenoids.

Try cutting down on meat, and see if this relieves the inflammation. Some people with joint pain believe that tomatoes, potatoes, aubergines and peppers increase inflammation.

PREMENSTRUAL SYNDROME (PMS)

Early in the perimenopause, some women start suffering PMS for the first time, or after a long time without it. Others experience similar symptoms of mood swings and tension, but at odd times of the month. Support your system with foods rich in vitamin B6 and magnesium.

Cut down on caffeine (in tea, coffee, cola drinks and chocolate), sugar and alcohol. Eat regularly, because low blood sugar exacerbates mood swings.

FATIGUE

A diet high in heavily processed foods can cause your blood-sugar levels to rise sharply and then fall, which has an exhausting effect. Filling up on fast foods also takes the place of more nutritious foods, leaving you undernourished even if overfed. And sometimes, when you're not making time for regular meals, you're simply tired because you're hungry.

HEAVY BLEEDING

As the perimenopause continues, many women find their periods becoming heavier, draining them of the iron that's carried in blood. Eating more iron-rich food is important to prevent anaemia, and the easiest form for your body to use is in meat (especially liver), fish or eggs. Have it with vegetables and salads, or a glass of orange juice. These are rich in vitamin C, which helps your body absorb the iron.

Don't drink tea or coffee within an hour of eating, as they stop you absorbing iron. And avoid bran, as it rushes food through your body before you have time to absorb all the nutrients.

Do soy foods help or harm?

Foods made from soybeans provide a low-fat form of protein. Soybeans are widely used in China, Japan and South-east Asia. In recent years their popularity has spread to Western countries too, first among vegetarians and lately among women approaching the menopause.

Vegetable foods can provide small amounts of a plant-based form of oestrogen called phytoestrogens. Soybeans are unusual in being rich in all kinds of phytoestrogens, especially the kind that has been found most similar to human oestrogen, called isoflavones.

Soy foods are now promoted as offering a replacement for oestrogen in a safer form than HRT. Asian women have fewer menopausal symptoms, we're told, and also have a lower risk of breast cancer.

But more recently critics have raised concerns about soy's effects on women who have breast cancer, or are in a high-risk group for developing it. They are concerned that the isoflavones could be all too similar to oestrogen, in that they too could cause tumours to grow. Some research has suggested that long-term use of phytoestrogen supplements (much more concentrated than in food) may thicken the endometrium (womb lining). This could be a precursor to endometrial cancer.

One recent study has even suggested that eating a lot of tofu could reduce the brain's function in old age. But, as with the cancer fears, there's not yet enough evidence to decide if this is right or not. The Indonesian elders who were studied could have relied on tofu because they could not afford other foods, for example, and their condition could result from the privations of poverty rather than from a specific food.

Critics have also said that soy may increase the risk of thyroid disease. This is true, but only in a specific group of people.

Research has shown that eating a lot of soy-based food could cause a goitre – a distinctive swelling in the throat. This would probably only happen to women who already have an underactive thyroid (which may not have been previously diagnosed). It is more likely in women whose diets are lacking in iodine.

Women living in Western countries aren't likely to be short of iodine, as there's plenty in dairy produce and seafood. If you're a vegan, refusing any kind of animal produce, you may be at risk. Iodine deficiency used to be a problem in some areas far from the sea, but the majority of countries where this was the case now add iodine to salt.

What about the benefits enjoyed by East Asian women? It's true that they are less likely to develop breast cancer than women in Europe, North America and other Westernized countries. However, their lifestyle is so different that you can't just pick out one factor. Traditionally, Asian women have been slim, physically active non-smokers, who eat much less meat than in the West and rarely drink alcohol. All these factors reduce the risk of breast cancer, so it's hard to say how much effect the soybeans are having. When East Asian women move to Western countries and take up our eating habits, their breast-cancer risk increases, along with their weight and their likelihood of smoking.

The facts are even harder to unravel for menopausal symptoms. Traditionally – in both Asia and the West – women rarely spoke about the menopause or anything else to do with their sexual health. If they did confide their problems, it was more likely to be in friends of the same age than in their daughters, so knowledge was rarely transmitted to the next generation. Even less was committed to print, so their experiences died with them. This was true in the West until the mid-twentieth century, and it remains largely true in Asia. So it's difficult to say how much a serene middle-aged Chinese or Japanese woman is enjoying the benefits of a soy-based diet and how much she is simply putting a good face on things.

Soy foods don't work for everyone. As in so many areas to do with hormones, some women's bodies are more sensitive than others to certain effects. And if what you took to be symptoms of the perimenopause were actually caused or exacerbated by an underactive thyroid (see Chapter 5 on midlife health), soy foods could make them worse.

However, there is more evidence in favour of soy than against it, including studies published in orthodox medical journals. Medical researchers have found that women who eat plenty of soy-based food actually have a lower risk of various cancers, including breast and thyroid cancers.

In particular, soy might protect against conditions that women face after the menopause. Soy-based foods may help strengthen bones, reducing the risk of osteoporosis. They protect the heart in numerous ways such as helping to reduce cholesterol levels. They reduce the risk of diabetes by stabilizing blood-sugar levels.

But the main reason women turn to soy-based foods is to relieve menopausal symptoms. Although there is not a lot of published evidence, many women say that soy helps reduce mood swings, brain fog, breast pain and even hot flushes – one of the most difficult symptoms to prevent.

Two new ways of taking soy are as supplements and as products such as margarines and burgers. However, supplements don't contain all the nutrients found in a whole food. And the long-term effects of modern soy products isn't yet known, because they haven't been around very long.

The best way to eat soy is as it's been enjoyed for centuries in the East, in the form of tofu (bean curd), edamame beans, or fermented soy products such as miso, natto and tempeh. (Soy sauce doesn't contain enough isoflavones to count.) If you'd like to try this Eastern alternative:

▶ *Start with about 20 mg of isoflavones a day, which is about one small serving of tofu or bowl of miso soup. Soy is high in protein and can replace a serving of meat.*

- ▶ If your symptoms haven't shown any improvement after a few weeks, gradually increase your intake to 40–80 mg a day, as long you feel well on it.
- ▶ Some people find any kind of legumes hard to digest. An enzyme product such as Beano may help.
- ▶ Vegans should get their doctor to check their iodine levels before switching to a high-soy diet. Don't take iodine supplements (including kelp tablets) before you know what you need, as overdosing could have long-term harmful effects.
- ▶ If you have been diagnosed with an oestrogen-dependent cancer such as breast cancer, or with thyroid disease, check with your doctor before starting to eat a lot of soy-based foods.
- ▶ Other rich sources of phytoestrogens include nuts, seeds (especially flax or linseed), legumes and wholegrain cereals.

> **Top tip**
> Take care of your thyroid by eating soy and sea vegetables together, as the Japanese do. Seaweeds such as kelp, dulse, hijiki and nori (laver) are rich in iodine.

A healthy weight and shape

It really is worth staying at a healthy weight. Being overweight sharply increases the number and severity of hot flushes. The less weight you put on painful joints, the less they hurt. Excess weight also speeds up the damage arthritis causes to joints.

A healthy weight is even more valuable over the long term, as postmenopausal weight gain steeply increases the risk of diseases including several cancers. A huge American study (Nurses' Health Study) found that women who gained 10 kg, or 22 lbs, after the menopause were 18 per cent more likely to suffer breast cancer. But those who lost that much weight after the menopause reduced their risk by 57 per cent.

Most women's bodies change shape to some extent during the perimenopause or soon after. We tend to accumulate an unhealthy type of fat on the abdomen, which increases the risk of heart disease and some cancers. So we're advised not to let our waist measurement reach more than 31.5 inches (80 cm), or more than 80 per cent of our hip measurement.

On the other hand, if you're too thin, your risk of osteoporosis is increased. Your bones may become brittle and porous, putting you at risk of fractures.

The body mass index (BMI) is a rough estimate of whether you are a healthy weight. It's not perfect, as it doesn't take account of the fact that muscle weighs more than fat. That's why, as you get fitter, you may not lose as much weight as you expect. But you're building healthy, firm muscle, which not only does you good but looks good too.

To find your BMI, go to the BBC's calculator at http://tinyurl.com/7yqp3. Or divide your weight in kilos (kg) by the square of your height in metres (m). So if you're 1.65 m tall and weigh 57 kg, your BMI is 57 divided by (1.65 × 1.65=) 2.72, which comes to just under 21.

Or multiply your weight in pounds by 700 and divide it by the square of your height in inches. So if you're 5 ft 5 in tall and weight 9 stone, or 126 pounds, that's (126 × 700 =) 88,200, divided by (65 × 65 =) 4225: just under 21.

A BMI under 19 is considered to be underweight, over 25 is overweight and over 30 is obese. Between 19 and 25 is healthy.

Summary

Healthy eating is more important than ever at this time of life, when the body's systems are starting to need a bit more support.

Cutting out junk food is almost as useful as eating and drinking more of the natural foods that our bodies are made to run on. Keeping to a healthy weight strongly reduces the risk of conditions such as arthritis and breast cancer. But it's not just about a generally healthy diet, valuable though that is. Certain nutrients are particularly effective in combating individual symptoms. Choose low-GI foods that help to keep blood-sugar levels stable. Don't expect foods to have the same sudden effects as drugs, though. Eating the right foods works slowly and powerfully over the long term.

Action plan: eating your symptoms away

1 *For two weeks, write down everything you eat and drink each day, no matter how small. Resist the temptation to be healthier than usual! It's worth finding out exactly what your eating patterns are.*
2 *Look through the list to see if you need to make any changes. If you do, and especially if you wish to lose weight, see if there's anything on the list that you don't particularly like and may just eat out of habit. If it's at the peak of the healthy eating pyramid, or not there at all, why not cut it out?*
3 *Cut down on sugar. Alcohol is high in sugar and also affects women's hormones, so if you're having any symptoms try keeping it down to a maximum of one unit a day.*
4 *Start replacing processed foods with fresh vegetables wherever possible.*
5 *Don't cook enough food to have second helpings, except of vegetables and salads.*
6 *Add individual foods to address any symptoms you are encountering.*

10 THINGS TO REMEMBER

1 Food can affect your hormones in both good and bad ways.

2 Eating nutritious food can improve your overall health to the level where any hormonal symptoms cause little problem. And certain individual ingredients may alleviate specific symptoms.

3 Some items may exacerbate hormonal problems, for example by destabilizing blood-sugar levels. Cutting down on sweets, fast foods and snacks should help.

4 If you only make one change to your diet at this time, eat more vegetables. These should form the basis of any eating plan, but especially now.

5 Hormonal changes put pressure on the digestive system during the perimenopause. Give it a hand by avoiding foods you find hard to digest and not eating late at night.

6 If you have a health condition or special dietary needs, you should check with your doctor before making any changes.

7 Phytoestrogens, contained in foods such as soybeans, may have a beneficial effect on hormones during and after menopause. But until more is known, it is wise not to use them if you have a hormone-dependent cancer.

8 Isoflavone supplements provide phytoestrogens in levels you couldn't get from any food, so their effects may be excessive.

9 Your needs are likely to change slightly between the start of perimenopause and the post-menopausal years.

10 The easy-to-follow eating plan in this book aims to address women's needs during perimenopause and after menopause, but is healthy and safe for people of any age.

13

Fitness

In this chapter you will learn:
- *what exercises work best at relieving different symptoms*
- *how to avoid the injuries most often suffered by women over 40*
- *why adding a fitness routine to your schedule actually gives you more time.*

Exercise is one of the most proven ways of relieving the symptoms of menopause, both mental and physical. It also improves all-round health so effectively that doctors consider it the best thing you can do apart from giving up smoking. It's an invigorating activity that makes life a lot more enjoyable, increasing your everyday vitality.

> ▶ *Studies have shown that exercise is a highly effective remedy for the vasomotor symptoms. It has been proved to reduce the number and severity of hot flushes and night sweats. For many women, it's better than HRT.*
> ▶ *The mood-lifting effects of exercise are well known. You're almost guaranteed to feel happier and more relaxed after a long walk or an aerobics class. It evens out mood swings and restores your equilibrium when you're going through a trying time.*
> ▶ *But did you know it also improves memory and other cognitive functions? This proves that the emotional lift it brings isn't just psychological but has a direct effect on the brain. In fact, physical fitness improves brain function*

so much that it's been shown to reduce the risk of dementia as you get older.

▶ *Aches and pains are partly caused by loss of the oestrogen that protects the muscles. But they're very much exacerbated by the kind of sedentary life many of us slip into about this time. Regular exercise relieves pain and protects the back and joints.*

▶ *Skin becomes dry and fragile as oestrogen levels fall. Exercise helps to replenish it with an increased supply of oxygenated blood.*

These are just a few of the powerful effects exercise has on menopausal symptoms. Exercise can be free, has virtually no side effects and is available to everyone.

In addition to its immediate benefits, exercise also combats the deterioration caused by ageing. It reduces the risk of almost all the most feared conditions of middle age and beyond – including Alzheimer's, heart disease, osteoporosis, diabetes and many cancers.

If a fitness programme seems hard to fit into your busy schedule, you may be surprised. Getting fit could give you so much extra vitality that you complete other tasks faster and have energy to take on more.

Warning

Be sure to consult your doctor before starting any new activity, especially if you have any health problems. Exercise is good for you, but launching into a strenuous new routine without adequate preparation could be harmful. Never ignore a pain or any new symptoms – especially those of heart disease, as described in Chapter 5 on midlife health – but seek medical advice. Listen to your body and do not try to push through pain.

Variety is the key to success

Different kinds of exercise target different functions. You need to do some of each kind for the best results. The best choice is something you enjoy that fits into your schedule, purely because you'll be more motivated to persevere with it.

> **Insight**
> A small amount of research and preparation pays large dividends in effectiveness, safety and enjoyment. Find a qualified instructor. Exercise on the correct surface, such as a sprung floor for aerobics. Make sure you're properly trained in any techniques and in use of any equipment. Always warm up before and cool down after exercising.

AEROBIC EXERCISE

This type of exercise speeds up your heart rate and improves your cardiovascular fitness, strengthening your heart, circulation and lungs. In the long term, this is essential to resist what are often called 'diseases' of old age but are actually just signs of deterioration, such as a weak heart and susceptibility to chest infections.

If you continue for more than about 20 minutes, you also start burning off fat.

You should exercise at a level where you're working up a sweat, but still just about able to keep a conversation going. Although it's good for the heart, if you have a heart condition, you should take your doctor's advice about what's safe for you.

Anything energetic will provide cardiovascular benefits. Safe and effective methods include:

▶ *aerobics: energetic dance-like exercises to music*
▶ *dancing*

- *brisk walking*
- *skipping (mind your knees)*
- *swimming.*

Insight

Some forms of exercise, though generally beneficial, may not suit you during this time. So fine-tune your workouts to meet your present needs. Avoid a strenuous aerobics class if you're bleeding heavily, for example, or a fast-moving team game if your co-ordination is affected.

RESISTANCE EXERCISE OR WEIGHT TRAINING

This is another important part of your fitness routine, specifically to build strength. It doesn't have to mean lifting weights: you're making your muscles work against some kind of resistance, and the most popular exercises use your own body weight.

We lose muscle strength rapidly after the menopause. Resistance exercise, to build and tone muscles, makes you stronger, faster and better able to avoid accidents. Strong muscles also hold your spine and joints more securely in place. As a bonus, muscle tissue gobbles up calories, helping to keep your weight down. And new research has shown that muscle strength is almost as valuable as cardiovascular fitness in promoting a long and healthy life.

Walking and dancing are good for the legs. But it's harder to strengthen the rest of the body in everyday life unless you're doing heavy work or often carrying shopping. Try the following:

- *Pilates, an exercise method using very finely honed movements to strengthen and protect muscles*
- *weight machines in a gym*
- *exercises with a rubber exercise band*
- *weight-training classes, or aerobics classes with a weight-training component at the end (ask for information at your local gym or leisure centre)*

- *home exercises such as sit-ups and triceps dips – these are easy to learn, preferably from a qualified instructor who can pick up any mistakes you may be making*
- *wearing wrist weights and doing arm exercises while walking may help.*

I felt better when I got back to the gym

'Exercise definitely helped with my mood swings,' says Sheila, a school assistant. She started running, and then going to a gym, while her children were growing up. Now 58, she works out four times a week and has the slim, toned body of a much younger woman.

'I used to get very bad mood swings, and I always knew when my period was due because I got really moody. My periods were so heavy I couldn't do anything, and I resented that. I'd feel a lot better as soon as I could get back to the gym again.'

FLEXIBILITY WORK

This type of exercise protects the muscles and keeps movements fluid and easy. As oestrogen levels decline, our muscles become more vulnerable to stiffness and damage. Stretching helps keep them supple, reducing the risk of injury and allowing joints their full range of movement. Stretch exercises help your muscles relax after a workout. Flexibility work also keeps you looking young when you move, instead of slipping into a stiff middle-aged gait. Good routines for promoting flexibility include:

- *yoga, the classic set of Indian stretch-and-twist exercises with a meditative background*

- *stretch classes, and stretch exercises at home or after any workout*
- *t'ai chi – a series of slow, flowing Chinese mind-and-body exercises, with fluid movements that promote suppleness*
- *qigong – individual exercises, also from China, aimed at moving and harnessing energy.*

WEIGHT-BEARING EXERCISE

This can be any of the exercises mentioned above. It should also be part of everyone's fitness routine, as it keeps your bones strong, reducing the risk of osteoporosis. It includes any exercise in which you carry the weight of your own body – that's most things except swimming, cycling and seated gym machines. It also includes resistance training, as the challenge to your muscles also challenges the nearest bones.

Walking is excellent for your legs and hips, but you also need to work your upper body or arms. Carrying shopping home would do this, but this is hard on your back if you have a heavy load. If you have any trouble with your back, do set exercises with a qualified trainer.

Try also:

- *walking on natural surfaces, where your legs and feet have to work more but are cushioned from impact*
- *yoga postures in which your muscles work to keep you in an unusual position*
- *trampolining or working on a rebounder*
- *step aerobics – a cardiovascular exercise class in which you're stepping on and off a small platform*
- *combining a walk with some upper-body exercises such as 'standing press-ups'. (Stand a short distance away from a wall, with your palms flat against it, then lean towards the wall and push yourself away. Engage your stomach muscles to prevent your back arching. Keep your spine straight and use the strength of your arms to move your body.)*

Exercise to meet your needs

In addition to the overall benefits of a fitness programme, different forms of exercise are useful for particular symptoms of the menopause. Otherwise, go for whatever you most enjoy, because this will motivate you to continue.

BALANCE

The effects of hormonal changes on the brain and central nervous system make many women clumsy during the perimenopause. In particular, women tend to trip easily, which can cause painful accidents and lead to long-term knee damage. If you're having a lot of trouble with this, activities such as walking or weight training with machines would be a safer option than fast-moving activities such as high-impact aerobics or team sports.

T'ai chi is the best exercise for improving balance, while also strengthening your legs to reduce the risk of falling. Yoga and Pilates also help; start out standing near a wall so you can use it as a support when you need to.

COORDINATION

If your hand-eye coordination is affected, making you misjudge distances and drop things, try throwing and catching a ball. Exercise works just as well for the brain as for the muscles, so you can actually train yourself to overcome the clumsiness caused by hormonal changes.

Playing tennis is an excellent way of keeping fit while improving coordination. If your balance is also affected, table tennis would be a safer place to start.

COGNITIVE FUNCTIONS

You may have been startled to realize that the hormonal changes of the menopause affected your brain, making you forgetful and unable to think of the right word. Luckily, the effects of exercise are just as surprising, but in a good way. Aerobic exercise increases the supply of oxygenated blood to all parts of your body, including the brain. And all parts, including the brain, show the good results.

Any activity in which you have to use tactics, such as paintballing, helps tone up the brain. The same is true when having to think on your feet, such as on an amusement-arcade dance machine. Dancing works on several levels, especially if you have to learn steps, as in Latin American, or follow instructions, as in a square dance or folk dance. You're getting excellent aerobic exercise, with the people around you motivating you to continue, even if you feel tired. Your brain has to work at learning the steps and your coordination – also involving the brain – is challenged by the fast movement.

Certain qigong exercises aim to stimulate the brain. The meditative effort involved in both t'ai chi and qigong helps retrain your mind to focus on what you're doing.

LEG STRENGTH

To avoid falls, you need to build strength in your legs as well as improving your balance. The legs are one of the easiest parts of the body to exercise, because they benefit from anything you do standing up: dancing, skipping, running and aerobics are just a few of the options. But if a tendency to trip over has reduced your confidence for fast-moving exercise, start out by doing safer strength work.

Working individual leg muscles on gym machines, with guidance from a member of staff, should bring good results. However, the easiest way to start is simply to spend more time walking. As your strength and balance improve, work up to walking on more challenging terrain such as hills. The quad and hamstring exercises detailed later in this chapter will also help.

MUSCLE PAIN

Don't be discouraged from muscle-building exercise if you're getting aches and pains in your limbs and back. Many women suffer these during the perimenopause, but stronger muscles are less susceptible to pain in the long run. Treat yourself to a massage every few weeks after you've been working out: many gyms have a sports-qualified massage therapist on the premises. Meanwhile, remember to do long, slow stretches to ease the muscles after working them or when they're aching.

Top tip

Hold a stretch for 20–30 seconds; less than 20 seconds won't have an effect, but hold it too long and you could cause injury. You should feel a gentle pull in the muscle, but not pain and not in the joint.

FLUID RETENTION

Both aerobic and muscle-building exercise help to squeeze excess fluid out of the tissues and move it along. A brisk walk every day works better than one big workout every week. Massage is very effective in getting the lymph system moving and flushing the extra fluid out of the body.

JOINT PAIN

To ease pain and prevent injury, you need to keep your joints supple as well as doing exercises for balance and leg strength. Yoga can overstretch sensitive joints, unless you have a very good instructor; therefore consider finding a trained yoga therapy teacher to make it work for you. Swimming is a useful non-weight-bearing exercise, but be aware that breaststroke can put a strain on your knees and neck.

MOOD SWINGS

If you're full of angry premenstrual energy, work it off with fast aerobics or running. Gardening may not officially count as exercise, but if you're leading a sedentary life you'd be surprised how much energy it uses. It's also been found to lift moods and relieve psychological disturbances. T'ai chi is deeply soothing and helps you to refocus your scattered energies.

FATIGUE

Aerobic exercise increases your vitality and energy. In a virtuous circle, this makes exercise easier and so you develop even more strength and energy. But if you're exhausted, you need to break into the circle somewhere easy. Yoga is very soothing, and if you keep to the beginner's level for as long as you need to, you can make progress without tiring yourself. If you have a hectic schedule, go for something you can easily do at home, but choose something you enjoy enough to motivate you, such as an easy-going dance DVD.

DEPRESSION

Fast-paced exercise causes your brain to produce hormones called endorphins, which make you feel good: the strongest motivation to exercise. This type of exercise works best with music, which has mood-lifting effects of its own. So get up and dance, take an aerobics class, or put your favourite music on headphones and go for a run – preferably somewhere without roads to cross.

STRESS

Eastern forms of exercise such as yoga, t'ai chi or qigong are designed to be calming, and there is plenty of published evidence showing that they help to reduce stress and its many harmful effects. T'ai chi has even been found to help people with diabetes control their blood-sugar levels, which are increased by stress. But you can also use any slow technique, such as muscle-building exercises, to still your racing thoughts. Practise them meditatively, focusing solely on what you're doing and letting all other thoughts float out of your mind.

VASOMOTOR SYMPTOMS

Yoga forward bends and inverted postures are claimed to have a balancing effect on hormones, and certainly yoga has been found to relieve hot flushes and night sweats. Building cardiovascular fitness also reduces the incidence of hot flushes. If you're suffering these a lot, you probably want to avoid anything that makes you feel hotter. In this case, aim to build your stamina through endurance exercise, such as long hikes, rather than anything fast-paced. Swimming is the ideal cooling exercise when you're feeling overheated.

A safe and effective inverted posture in yoga is 'Legs up the Wall'. To do this, lie on your side with your bottom close to the wall, then turn onto your back, without arching your spine, and stretch your legs up the wall.

HEAVY PERIODS

Any kind of gentle exercise will help relieve the congested feeling of a heavy period, and walking in peaceful surroundings is among the most gentle. T'ai chi and qigong are also helpful. Avoid anything strenuous that will make you feel even more drained.

INSOMNIA

Regular exercise is one of the most effective cures for insomnia. It has been shown to reduce the amount of time people take to drop off and increase both the number of hours they sleep and the amount of restorative deep sleep.

You just have to find the time of day that suits you best. Many people find that aerobic exercise in the evening wakes them up, in which case they should fit it in earlier in the day. This is most likely among beginners; as you become fitter, your body adapts more rapidly and you may well find you can sleep straight after a workout. Flexibility exercises, such as stretches, help you unwind before you go to bed.

Top tip

It's never too late to learn to swim. Ask at your local baths if there's a teacher experienced in teaching adults. Being able to put your face in the water gives you many more options.

Avoiding injury

One of the main reasons people give up a new fitness programme is because of injury. It's not usually a serious injury, just enough to keep them out of the gym and break the exercise habit. It is usually caused by launching enthusiastically into a new activity without adequate preparation.

The longer you continue, the fitter you'll become, the more you'll learn about exercising safely and effectively, and the less likely you'll be to suffer an injury.

Meanwhile, make a safe and successful start by:

▶ *wearing suitable shoes and clothing for what you're doing, including a well-fitting sports bra to protect your breasts*
▶ *ensuring your instructor is qualified and the space you're using is suitable. (For example, if you go to aerobics classes – especially if they're not low-impact – make sure they're on a proper sprung floor, as in a gym, and the teacher is RSA-qualified)*
▶ *informing your instructor if you have any injuries or weak spots, and asking them to warn you if there are any moves you shouldn't make*

- *learning how to use any equipment before you start. (If you're using machines in a gym, you should be given a training session by a qualified member of staff. Don't hesitate to ask questions if anything isn't clear)*
- *warming up at the beginning and cooling down at the end of every session*
- *starting at a comfortable level and increasing gently. (A safe rule of thumb is a maximum ten per cent increase a week in either intensity of effort, as measured, for example, by weight machines, or number of repetitions of an exercise, or amount of time spent exercising)*
- *stopping at once if you get a sharp pain. (If the pain is in your chest, seek medical help immediately. If a pain elsewhere hasn't worn off within three days, go to your doctor)*

Top tip

If you feel dizzy when bending forward, tell your GP because this could be a blood pressure problem. But if it's just caused by unfitness, ask your teacher for an adaptation. In yoga, for example, you can bend halfway using a table for support. As you get fitter, the dizziness should wear off.

Protect your knees

Along with backs, knees are the part of the body most likely to cause pain as you go through the menopause and beyond. Exercise has been proved to reduce the risk of becoming disabled, even if you already have arthritis in your knees. On the other hand, injuries increase a joint's risk of developing arthritis. And as knee arthritis is a very common problem for women over 50, it's well worth taking special care of these complicated joints.

This is partly because of the way we're made. There's a possibility that hormonal changes may affect the ligaments, including those that hold the knee in place. If so, the fluctuations of perimenopause may make the knees less stable than before or afterwards.

What's certain is that women have looser ligaments and more mobile kneecaps than men. We also have wider hips in relation to the length of our thighs. This creates a greater angle at the knee between thighbone and shinbone, which can make the kneecap slip outwards during movement, instead of staying neatly in the groove at the end of the thighbone.

A common problem for women is patellofemoral pain, or problems arising in the joint between the kneecap and the thighbone. This hurts when you're running, going up or down stairs or doing a step aerobics class. It may also make your knee click. It causes an ache behind the knee that makes you need to stretch your leg out when you've been sitting for a while.

A sudden twinge when you twist your knee may be from a damaged meniscus. These C-shaped cartilages act as shock absorbers, one on each side of the knee. The tissue becomes drier with age, so tears become more common as the menopause approaches. Other symptoms are clicking, locking or swelling.

The main problem seems to be the way we move. Instead of landing initially on our toes from a jump, we tend to put our feet down flat, and keep our legs straighter than men do when jumping or doing aerobics.

Ensure your exercise is suitable if you have any concerns about your knees. Activities to be careful of include those in which you change direction suddenly at speed. Team sports such as netball are hard on the knees, as you're likely to get bumped or knocked down. And running long distances or on hard pavements subjects knees to a constant jarring pressure.

There's no need to be timid, but it makes sense to take up an activity that's less likely to hurt. Try power-walking instead of running, for example, or low-impact aerobics instead of high-impact.

Many activities are kinder to your knees if you make some small adaptations. Cycling can put a strain on knees, which may be cured by adjusting the saddle height. Swimming is an excellent option, as your knees aren't carrying the weight of your body. However, the rotation-and-thrust movement of breaststroke can put stress on knee ligaments. So if you have trouble with your knees, try other styles such as crawl or backstroke too.

▶ *Learn to land safely from a jump, with your legs and hips bent to absorb the impact.*
▶ *Wear shoes specifically designed for your activity, and make sure you're training on the correct surface. Shoes that provide a lot of traction may improve performance, but they can also increase the risk of injury.*
▶ *If you've suffered an injury, swap to activities that don't involve twisting the knee, especially at speed, or putting it under undue pressure. Don't exercise when the joint is stiff, swollen or painful.*

BUILD SUPPORT FOR YOUR KNEES

A knee injury is one of the most common reasons for dropping out of exercise and a frequent cause of arthritis in later life. So it's worth taking extra care of the tendons and muscles that stabilize these joints. Doing some knee exercises every day at home will help build strength and stability for any kind of activity.

Both hamstrings (tendons at the back of the knee) and quadriceps (large muscles at the front of the thigh) play an important role, but become stiff and weak without exercise. The knee bend exercise helps correct the alignment of the leg.

Hamstring exercise
Stand with feet together, abdominal muscles engaged to prevent your back arching. Step forward with your right foot and bend both knees as if curtsying. Your step should be long enough to allow your right knee to bend without the kneecap going further forward than your toes, and your left heel should rise off the floor. Step back to the starting position and repeat with left leg. Do five repetitions on each leg, stopping if your knees start to hurt.

Hamstring stretch
Sit with one knee bent and the other leg extended along the floor in front of you, toes pointing to the ceiling. Lean forward until you feel a gentle stretch in the straight leg. Hold for a count of 20. Repeat twice on each leg.

Quadriceps exercise
Stand on one leg and bend the knee so you dip about six inches. Hold for a count of ten. Repeat ten times.

Quadriceps stretch
Stand with one hand on the wall for support. Lift one leg and pull your foot towards your buttocks. Hold for a count of 20, then release the foot and stand straight. Repeat twice on each leg.

Knee bend
Stand with your back against a wall, feet slightly away from the wall and hip-width apart. Lengthen your spine and engage your abdominal muscles and buttocks to stop the back arching. Check that your weight is evenly on both feet and bend your knees slowly. Keep the kneecaps in line with the second toe: don't let knees or ankles drop inwards or outwards. Hold for a count of 5–10. Return slowly to the starting position. Repeat twice.

Protect your pelvic floor

One of the most unwelcome symptoms of the menopause is urinary incontinence – accidentally losing some urine when you cough or laugh. (About one woman in five will also have encountered this after having her first child.) It's another sign of low oestrogen levels weakening muscles, in this case those that control the bladder.

Strenuous exercise or heavy lifting can exacerbate the problem. So even if your pelvic floor is fine at the moment, don't risk damaging it while you're working out. Even when doing exercises that are considered safe, such as curl-ups, you need to brace the pelvic-floor muscles against abdominal pressure. Otherwise, tightening abdominal muscles makes the pelvic floor bulge downwards. See Chapter 7 for Kegel exercises that strengthen the pelvic floor.

If it's so important to avoid injury, maybe I shouldn't be taking exercise!

Don't be put off by all these warnings. It is important to try to avoid injuries, especially to the joints, as these can be a nuisance in the long term. But even if you do have an accident, it's likely to be minor and far outweighed by the benefits of exercise.

Exercise actually saves you from having serious accidents, through building up strength, flexibility and balance. It may be menopausal lack of coordination that made you catch your foot on the kerb. But you tripped and fell because your legs didn't support you, your other foot couldn't move quickly enough and you were unable to regain balance in time. As you get fitter, this is less likely to happen.

Exercise confers so many other benefits in terms of overall health, strength and energy that, even if you're unlucky enough to be injured, you'll still be better off than before you started. And your improved health will help you heal much faster than an unfit person having a similar injury for other reasons.

Summary

Getting fit not only relieves or prevents symptoms of the menopause, it also improves your life in numerous other ways. It strengthens your heart (cardiovascular fitness), builds bones and muscles, increases flexibility, improves your balance and protects your brain. It reduces the risk of numerous diseases and conditions, including many that you wouldn't think had anything to do with physical fitness. And it delays the visible and internal signs of ageing. Hardly anything you do during the perimenopause can improve the quality of your life as much as regular exercise. If you need extra motivation, choose activities that are known to reduce the symptoms that are bothering you most. Take measures to reduce the risk of injury – although few injuries do as much harm as not exercising.

Action plan: building strength and energy to face all challenges

1 *Find out what activities are available in your area and choose some that look interesting. Try to include aerobic, muscle-building and flexibility work.*
2 *Try out several activities to find the ones that best meet your needs. Take part in taster classes wherever possible.*
3 *Work out a schedule you can stick to, with exercise as a high priority. Do a minimum of three 30-minute sessions a week, aiming towards five hours a week as an ideal.*
4 *If your motivation flags, go with a friend, join a group or take part in team activities: people help each other continue.*

10 THINGS TO REMEMBER

1 *Fitness strengthens your whole system, reducing the uncomfortable effects of menopausal symptoms.*

2 *If you're not very fit now, gaining fitness could have a beneficial effect on your hormones, reducing the fluctuations that cause symptoms such as mood swings.*

3 *Exercise itself (not just the resultant fitness) has been proved to relieve mild depression, nourish the skin, promote sleep, ease aches and pains, improve memory and help to keep weight under control.*

4 *Regular exercise reduces the risk of many diseases, including most of those that strike at midlife or later.*

5 *You can choose specific exercises to relieve your current symptoms and avoid those that could make them worse.*

6 *Even vasomotor symptoms – the hardest to control – may be eased, by certain yoga positions or endurance exercise such as long walks.*

7 *Declining oestrogen levels make joints and muscles more vulnerable. Exercise protects them in the long term, but take extra care to avoid injuries while you're getting fit.*

8 *Knees and back are especially easy to injure at this time. So follow the advice about these to make the most of your fitness routine without coming to harm.*

9 *Wear the right kind of shoes, correctly fitted, for whatever sport or exercise you're doing.*

10 *Check with your doctor before taking up any form of exercise, making sure the doctor knows if you have any health condition.*

14

Early and premature menopause

In this chapter you will learn:
- *why menopause may start earlier than expected*
- *how you can reduce the risk of this happening*
- *what to do if you discover it has started.*

The average age for a woman to have her last period naturally is about 51. But in some women it happens a lot earlier.

Premature menopause is when you stop having periods before the age of 40. This happens for various reasons, including illnesses and medical treatments. It's sometimes called 'premature ovarian failure' if it happens naturally. This could be a long-term result of things that happened in your childhood or even earlier, in the womb.

If you stop having periods in your early forties, it's known as early menopause. This doesn't necessarily mean there's anything wrong. It's just your individual body clock reaching this stage at the early end of the 'normal' spectrum. But occasionally it's a sign of something else that may need treatment.

An early or premature menopause can cause some problems. For a start, it means you stop being able to have children earlier than you would expect. And your body has to cope with conditions caused by a shortage of certain hormones sooner than usual.

It's worth noticing if any of these changes are happening in your body, so that you can take action, if you wish to, in good time.

If you suspect premature ovarian failure and you wish to have children, see a fertility specialist without delay. There is sometimes a chance that you still have usable eggs.

Premature menopause

About one woman in 100 will stop having periods before she reaches 40. As well as unavoidable conditions, anything that damages your ovaries can trigger a premature menopause. This can include illness and hospital treatment.

> **Insight**
> Premature menopause is also known as premature ovarian failure (POF).

Premature ovarian failure doesn't always mean you can't still get pregnant. In some cases, although the ovaries aren't working as before, there are still eggs available.

There are several reasons for premature menopause.

▶ **Illness** – *More than 20 per cent of women who undergo premature menopause have an autoimmune condition of some kind. Many have some form of thyroid disease, or type 1 diabetes – the sort you are born with rather than develop in later life. It is now thought that certain childhood illnesses may destroy some of the eggs in the womb. Mumps, for example, has long been known to possibly reduce a boy's later fertility; now it seems it may also affect some girls. Serious diseases such as tuberculosis and malaria can have the same effect.*
▶ **Family history** – *It could stem from genetic reasons, if any of your relatives have had the same experience.*
▶ **Pre-birth events** – *Because you're born with your entire lifetime's supply of eggs already inside you, they could be affected by your experiences in the womb. Some babies are simply born with very few eggs, possibly because their mother*

caught a viral infection during the pregnancy. For some reason, premature menopause is five times more common among twins, whether they're identical or not.

▶ **Medical treatment** – *Certain medicines can bring on a premature menopause. These tend to be life-saving treatments, notably chemotherapy for cancer. Radiotherapy for cancer may have the same effect.*

▶ **Lifestyle** – *Factors such as smoking and being underweight wouldn't be enough to cause premature menopause by themselves, but they add to the pressure on your ovaries.*

▶ **Surgery** – *A hysterectomy (removal of the uterus) normally stops your periods at once. However, if you still have working ovaries, you should not be menopausal: in theory, your body should still produce the hormones appropriate to your age. In reality, the operation may restrict blood flow to the ovaries and cause them to stop working sooner, bringing an early menopause. As hysterectomy is often carried out for conditions that aren't life threatening, such as fibroids or a prolapsed womb, it's worth looking into alternatives. If you're having a hysterectomy, ensure that your ovaries aren't removed unless this is essential for your health. Losing your ovaries will cause immediate menopause, as your main source of oestrogen will have gone. Removal of one ovary increases the risk that menopause will come early. Other kinds of abdominal surgery may also damage blood supply to the ovaries, though that's less likely than after a hysterectomy.*

Insight

If your ovaries are removed, you will immediately experience menopause. Ovaries are usually only removed by themselves if they are diseased. But they are also sometimes taken when the womb is removed, which may not be necessary for your health. If you are having a hysterectomy for any reason other than cancer, ask your doctor if your ovaries can be kept in place.

Top tip

Lack of periods isn't a sure sign of menopause, but may indicate other problems. See your doctor for a check-up.

Early menopause

If you have your last period before the age of 45, it is considered to be early.

> **Insight**
> Early menopause is a lot more common than premature menopause.

One of the main predictors is the number of periods you have had. If you've never been pregnant, or have cycles shorter than 28 days, or don't take the contraceptive Pill (which prevents ovulation), you are likely to reach menopause earlier.

However, that's only if you've used up your eggs through natural causes. It is no longer thought that assisted-fertility techniques such as in-vitro fertilization (IVF) cause early menopause, even though they use up numerous eggs. And if you've ever stopped having periods at any time for unhealthy reasons (see below), you are at higher risk of an early menopause.

The main difference between early and premature menopause, apart from those five years, is that early menopause often stems from lifestyle factors. This means you can take action to prevent it.

- ▶ **Smoking** – *This brings menopause forward by about two years. As this is an average, it means that some smokers have even fewer years of reproductive life.*
- ▶ **Chemical exposure** – *The modern world is heavily polluted by endocrine-disrupting xenoestrogens, chemicals that mimic some effects of oestrogen. These are produced as a by-product of industrial processes and are so widespread that they have been found to change the sex of fish in rivers. As with everything to do with hormones, some people are more sensitive to them than others. As they are known to disrupt hormonal processes, they have been linked by some researchers to infertility and early menopause.*

- ▶ **Depression** – *Women who have been treated for depression are likely to enter menopause earlier. It's not known whether this is because their low moods affected their hormones, or the other way round, or whether it's another side effect of antidepressant drugs.*
- ▶ **Malnutrition** – *Beware of a highly processed modern diet. Even 'enriched' products don't contain enough added nutrients to replace the huge number lost through processing. Social researchers have found that women who have lived through hard times, whether in childhood or later life, start the menopause earlier. Modern poverty, in the developed world at least, is linked not with lack of food but with junk food, containing few essential nutrients other than calories.*
- ▶ **Weight** – *Being heavily overweight can bring your menopause forward, but so can being very underweight. Try to keep to a healthy size.*
- ▶ **Anything that stops your periods unnaturally** – *Losing too much body fat can do this. It can happen through overexercising as well as crash dieting. Shocks, depression and stress can also stop your periods. These unnatural breaks – unlike natural events such as pregnancy – seem to damage the system and bring menopause on earlier.*

Insight

Having your womb removed (hysterectomy) stops your periods, but doesn't necessarily cause the hormonal changes of menopause, as long as your ovaries aren't removed at the same time. However, like any abdominal surgery, it may bring menopause a little earlier than expected, by damaging the ovaries or the blood flow to them.

How do I know if my menopause is starting early?

If you're hoping to have children, it's important to know how fast your body clock is ticking. But even if you don't, an early menopause brings forward the risk of old-age diseases. It's not always obvious what's happening, and finding out where you stand could prevent you taking the wrong course of action.

It's often thought that the first sign of perimenopause – the changes leading up to menopause – is when your periods become irregular or infrequent. For many women, this is not the case. You may still go on having periods for a while when your ovaries are failing, as you can have a period without having ovulated.

You may even ovulate occasionally. This would mean that you haven't run out of eggs, but something is preventing your ovaries working normally. When you're having periods, you wouldn't usually know if you have ovulated or not.

When you stop taking the contraceptive pill in your thirties, it may take a year or more for your cycles to return to normal. Blood tests done during this time may tell you, incorrectly, that you've started the perimenopause.

Changes to look out for include the following:

▶ **perimenopausal symptoms** *such as hot flushes, even if your periods are still normal*
▶ **new menstrual problems** *such as painful periods or PMS – this could be a sign of perimenopause, if you either hadn't had them before or you had stopped having them long ago*
▶ **irregular or missed periods,** *if yours have always been regular in the past. Remember that these alone aren't evidence of perimenopause, and conversely you could be in perimenopause with perfectly regular periods.*

Natural family planning or fertility control can also provide clues as to whether perimenopause has started. This involves observing your body's changes such as daily temperature and consistency of secretions at the time of ovulation. It's used either as a natural form of contraception or to improve chances of conceiving a child. But whether you're concerned about fertility or not, it also gives you some insight into your hormonal processes.

Hormone tests

If you think you may be experiencing early or premature menopause, consider having hormone tests to give you some idea what's happening. For most of your reproductive life, you mainly produce follicle-stimulating hormone (FSH) during the first week of the monthly cycle and luteinizing hormone (LH) around the time of ovulation. Levels of FSH and LH increase throughout the perimenopause, while oestrogen and progesterone decrease. If the LH level is high in relation to the FSH, this could be a sign of another hormonal condition such as polycystic ovaries, which can cause some of the same symptoms as perimenopause.

Don't rely on these tests, though, as hormone levels can fluctuate wildly in the early stages of perimenopause. A couple of normal readings could provide false reassurance.

In the future, scientific advances may be able to give you more help, but tests are unlikely to be available soon. Ultrasound may be able to tell how many eggs you have left, but not what condition they're in. Researchers are working on drugs that they hope will slow down the rate at which eggs are used.

Scientists are currently trying to develop a blood test to measure the level of anti-Müllerian hormone (AMH), which is involved in the development of ovarian follicles. If all goes well, they hope eventually to be able to tell a woman when she is likely to reach menopause. But it's early days yet, and although predictive tests can be helpful they rarely provide pinpoint accuracy.

Can it be delayed?

Premature menopause stems largely from factors you can't control. But there are a few you can influence, the most important being abdominal surgery. Fortunately, less intrusive treatments have become available for many gynaecological conditions. So if you have a condition that's not life threatening, ask your doctor about gentler alternatives. These are detailed in *Hysterectomy: is it right for you?* by Janet Wright (Sheldon, 2009). See the 'Taking it further' section for some helpful groups.

If you're at risk of an early menopause, there are steps you can take to at least delay it. These also ease any additional pressure towards premature menopause. And whether you're at risk or not, they can do you, and your hormones, nothing but good.

- ▶ *Stop smoking.*
- ▶ *Cut down on alcohol, if you are drinking more than a couple of units a day.*
- ▶ *Improve the quality of your life by reducing stress, doing things that make you happy and taking time to relax.*
- ▶ *Avoid hormone-disrupting chemicals as far as possible by eating organic foods, using natural materials rather than plastics, never using artificial chemicals in your house or garden, and avoiding dry-cleaners.*

Top tip

You can still get pregnant when you're not having periods, so you should use contraception if you don't wish to, until menopause is confirmed. If you're taking HRT, try barrier methods of contraception such as condoms or the cervical cap.

What if it has already happened?

If you have definitely reached the menopause, you should consider replacing the oestrogen your ovaries are no longer providing. Doctors generally advise using hormone replacement therapy until you're about 50. If you've had a hysterectomy, this will be oestrogen-only HRT. But if you still have your womb, you'll need to take progestogen too, to protect the womb lining from cancer.

Taking HRT after an early or premature menopause is intended to delay conditions such as heart disease and osteoporosis, which become increasingly common after the menopause. Although an early menopause does increase your risk of some diseases, little research has been done on the relative risks and benefits of drugs such as HRT for women below 45.

Early menopause may actually reduce your risk of blood clots and breast cancer – two of the main concerns raised by taking HRT. So taking HRT to bring your oestrogen level back to that of most women at your age may only readjust your risk to normal.

Insight

Doctors are increasingly reluctant for women to stay on HRT for more than five years because of the health risks. This is something to discuss with your health specialist, and keep under review as new information becomes available. Meanwhile, ensure you have regular mammograms and other recommended health checks.

Lifestyle changes, including diet and exercise, play a major role in promoting good health and wellbeing at any time of life. Many women only make such changes after the menopause, when they're already in their fifties and starting to tire easily. You have the advantage of your youthful energy to build a lifestyle that could make your life even better than before the menopause. See earlier chapters for more details.

- ▶ *Take regular weight-bearing exercise to protect your bones from osteoporosis.*
- ▶ *Eat healthily to reduce your risk of other diseases you may encounter after the menopause.*
- ▶ *Create life-enhancing habits to carry you through any challenging times.*

Sudden menopause

A sudden shock can stop your periods. This can result from either an emotional blow, such as bereavement or relationship breakdown, or a physical trauma such as an accident or operation. This can happen at any age, and if your periods don't start again within a few months, it should be investigated. But if you're close to the age at which you would have started perimenopausal changes anyway, the shock can trigger the menopause.

If you're over 45, this doesn't count as early or premature menopause. But people age at different rates, and your body has its own internal clock. If your menopause is triggered by a sudden shock, you could be at risk of some of the problems faced by women whose menopause has arrived at an earlier age.

If you hadn't previously had much sign of the perimenopause, tell your doctor what has happened and ask about hormone tests. Your hormone levels may remain unbalanced for some time as your body tries to adjust to the unexpected change. This could increase your risk of certain diseases including cancers, so you should keep an eye on any changes.

It all seemed to freeze up inside

'I never went through a perimenopause,' says Maria, who is now 56. 'My periods were starting to get lighter, but still came every 28 days like clockwork. Then a good friend of mine, who was younger than me, died very suddenly when

I was 50, and I was so shocked and upset, it all seemed to freeze up inside. I never had another period. After that I got a few hot flushes, or I should say warm flushes, nothing much.

'I'd stopped having periods a couple of times in the past, once when I was going through a difficult patch when I was working abroad, and once after an operation. They came back after a few months each time. I suppose this time I was nearer the end of it anyway, so they just didn't bother. I make sure I never miss my mammograms now, because apparently you can be left with your hormones in a mess when you stop menstruating so suddenly.'

Summary

A small number of women experience early (before the age of 45) or premature (before 40) menopause. This can be caused by surgery such as hysterectomy or by unavoidable factors such as genetics or childhood illness. An unhealthy lifestyle can also bring menopause earlier. You can slow down the process to some extent by healthy living, which can also improve your hormonal health generally. But you cannot prevent premature ovarian failure. You may still become pregnant even without periods, while your ovaries haven't completed shutting down. Doctors usually recommend HRT until the age at which most women reach the menopause, about 50.

Action plan: dealing with an unexpected change

1   *If you suspect you are at risk of early or premature menopause, ask around your family. You may find this has happened to*

aunts or other older relatives. Also look into your own medical history, with the help of your parents and your doctor.

2 If the menopause has come early, ask your doctor if it's possible to find out why, and have tests for conditions that may be related. This could be a chance to diagnose and treat another condition.

3 In reading about the risks of HRT, including the chapter in this book, keep in mind that most of the evidence relates to older women. Health risks and benefits may be different for women who reach the menopause at an early age. Keep up to date with new research if you can.

4 Take action recommended by your health specialists – and in Chapters 11, 12 and 13 on lifestyle, nutrition and fitness – to support your health and reduce your disease risks naturally.

10 THINGS TO REMEMBER

1 *If your periods stop permanently before the age of 40, this is premature menopause, also known as premature ovarian failure (POF).*

2 *Affecting about one woman in 100, POF is usually caused by medical or genetic reasons and cannot be delayed.*

3 *If your periods stop before the age of 45, this is called early menopause and is much more common than POF. It often stems from lifestyle factors.*

4 *If you've had children, or your cycles are longer than 28 days, or you're on the contraceptive Pill (which prevents ovulation), your risk of early menopause is reduced. The fewer eggs you've used through natural causes, the less likely menopause is to come early.*

5 *The sooner you reach menopause, the earlier your risk of developing any of the diseases that become more common afterwards.*

6 *However, early or premature menopause may reduce your risk of breast cancer and blood clots.*

7 *If you suspect menopause is starting early, you can have hormone tests to check, but these aren't always reliable.*

8 *Ultrasound may show how many eggs you have left, but not whether they're in good enough condition for a successful pregnancy.*

9 *Pregnancy can occur during the months after periods have stopped, as you may still ovulate for a while. It's rare but possible.*

10 *Asking older relatives when they had their final period can give you a warning if it tends to be early. Don't be too reassured if it's not early, as individual factors also play a part.*

Taking it further

Products
- *Cool Sleepwear* *www.coolsleepwear.co.uk*
- *Chillow* *www.soothsoftshop.co.uk/chillow.php*

Other help and advice
- *The British Association of Behavioural and Cognitive Psychotherapies, www.babcp.com maintains a register of practitioners.*
- *Daisy Network Premature Menopause Support Group, daisy@daisynetwork.org.uk, www.daisynetwork.org.uk*
- *NHS Direct, www.nhsdirect.nhs.uk, and nurse-led UK telephone advice line Tel: 0845 46 47.*
- *Women's Health Concern, helpline (UK) Tel: 0845 123 2319 www.womens-health-concern.org*

Complementary therapies
- Traditional Herbal Medicines – a guide to their safer use *(Hammersmith Press) by Lakshman Karalliedde and Indika Gawarammana.*
- *Natural Health Advisory Service www.naturalhealthas.com Tel: (UK) 01273 609699.*
- *Women to Women www.womentowomen.com Tel: (US) 1-800-798-7902.*

Nutrition
- *The George Mateljan Foundation – www.whfoods.com. For solid scientific but easy-to-read information about food and nutrition.*
- *thefoody.com/basic/vegseason.html. Find out what foods are in season locally and how to cook them, with recipes.*

Exercise

▶ *Yoga Biomedical Trust www.yogatherapy.org*
   Tel: (UK) 020 7689 3040.
▶ *British Wheel of Yoga www.bwy.org.uk*
   Tel: (UK) 01529 306851.

Appendix: understanding the research

Why are there so many conflicting reports about the risks, or benefits, of HRT, as mentioned in Chapter 8?

Opponents of all things orthodox have long claimed that drug trials funded by the drug companies only showed what the manufacturers wanted them to show. This didn't have a lot of credibility, as some of the opponents were themselves selling unproven remedies. However, during the past few years many academic studies and investigative reports have backed this claim to some extent (see HRT and the drug companies below).

Studies that are funded by charities or the government may be more reliable. The UK's Million Women Study is funded by the National Health Service (NHS), the charity Cancer Research UK and the Medical Research Council. The Women's Health Initiative (WHI) is funded by the US National Institutes of Health.

Factors affecting the outcome

The way a study is set up can make a difference to its results.

A 'randomized controlled trial' is one in which volunteers agree to take a treatment, often a tablet of some sort. They are assigned to different groups, one group taking the tablets and the other not. They are assigned randomly to try to ensure that the two groups are as similar as possible.

If this randomized trial is 'placebo-controlled', it means one group is taking a placebo, or pretend treatment (usually a plain pill).

If it's a 'double-blind' placebo-controlled trial, no one, including the people providing the pills, knows until the end who is taking the real treatment and who is taking the placebo. At the end, the results for the two groups are compared to see how well the treatment worked.

An 'observational' trial is one in which researchers simply look at what people are doing, without asking them to make any changes. Many of the studies in which HRT was found to be useful have been observational.

Parts of the WHI study were randomized controlled trials; other parts were observational.

The Million Women Study was purely observational. It recruited all its volunteers through the NHS breast-screening programme. All women in the UK are invited to have a mammogram every three years after they reach the age of 50. The 1.3 million women who took part simply answered questions, over the years, about their health, lifestyle and the medicines they took. Half of them had never tried HRT.

The sort of people involved in a trial can make a difference to its results. Unlike most drugs, HRT is made for people who aren't ill. Healthy people who volunteer to take part in a study may well be more active, more clued-up about health, more likely than average to have a good outcome generally.

Some studies have shown that doctors and other educated women, who eat a good diet and take care of their health, have been the most likely to use HRT. These are the sort of women who tend to have the best health anyway. American researchers found in 2004, for example, that HRT users were more likely than non-users to drink less than one unit of alcohol a day, know their cholesterol level and consider themselves to be in good health. They found that heavily overweight and physically inactive women were the least likely to use HRT.

Some experts say this 'healthy user' effect may help to explain why HRT seems to do better in observational studies than in independent drug trials. Researchers have noted, for example, that elderly women who used HRT tend to have better teeth, and lose fewer, than their contemporaries who didn't use it. Some think that this is because oestrogen protects the teeth in the same way as it protects the bones. But, as previous studies have found HRT users to be generally more active in looking after their health, it could also be because they take care of their teeth too.

Although all British women are invited to have a mammogram when they reach 50, those who do attend (from whom all the 1.3 Million Women were recruited) may be healthier than the general population, as they are more conscientious about their health. If this did affect the results, it would skew them in favour of HRT, not against it.

ABSOLUTE AND RELATIVE RISK

Finally, some critics have complained that studies have exaggerated the dangers of HRT by expressing their results as relative risk rather than absolute risk.

Absolute risk means your chance of ever developing a particular disease during a particular period. Your absolute lifetime risk of breast cancer, for example, is that one-in-eight-women figure we've often heard quoted.

Relative risk compares one risk with another, for example comparing your risk of developing breast cancer if you take HRT against your risk of developing it if you don't take HRT. The WHI trial was stopped early after it found that taking combined HRT increased a woman's risk of breast cancer by 26 per cent among other dangers. But that increased the risk from 0.30 per cent each year for women who didn't take HRT to 0.38 per cent for those who did. In absolute terms, it meant that taking HRT increases a woman's risk of developing breast cancer by 0.08 per cent a year.

However, relative risk is the measure used by most scientific studies – including the drug trials that have shown the benefits of HRT. If the WHI or Million Women studies had switched to measuring only absolute risk, they could not have been compared with the existing research on a like-for-like basis. It would be difficult to compare the effects of treatments (or of not using a treatment) without expressing them as relative risks.

So, if the dangers of HRT have been exaggerated, the benefits have been exaggerated in exactly the same way.

Details of the recent studies

One of the WHI trials had 16,000 women taking either combined HRT (oestrogen and progestogen) or a placebo. Ten thousand other women, who had previously had a hysterectomy, took part in a separate trial in which the active drug was oestrogen only. This was because oestrogen alone was already known to cause womb cancer.

The WHI was looking at the long-term results of HRT use in women aged 50–79 who no longer had periods. At the time it was set up, in the 1990s, long-term use of HRT was hoped to protect against heart disease, stroke and possibly other diseases of old age. But the combined-HRT trial was stopped early in 2002 because it was found to increase the risk of breast cancer, slightly increase the risk of heart disease, and overall do more harm than good. The oestrogen-only trial was also stopped early, in 2004, because it showed no benefit for heart disease and increased the risk of a stroke.

The WHI research found that women taking combined HRT had the following increased risks, in comparison with those taking a placebo: they were 41 per cent more likely to have a stroke, 29 per cent more likely to have a heart attack, 111 per cent more likely to have a blood clot, 22 per cent more likely to have any kind of cardiovascular disease and 26 per cent more likely to have breast cancer. On the other hand, those taking combined HRT were 37 per cent less likely to have bowel cancer, 33 per cent less likely to have a hip fracture and 24 per cent less likely to have any kind of fracture.

These are percentages of very small percentages. In almost all cases, an individual woman had less than a one per cent risk, in any year, of getting any of those conditions. A 41 per cent increase in the risk of a stroke, for example, meant the risk increased from 0.21 per cent of participants to 0.29 per cent. A 26 per cent increase in breast-cancer risk raised it from 0.30 per cent to 0.38 per cent for any one woman in a year.

On the other hand, very large numbers of women take HRT. The WHI results meant that out of every million postmenopausal women on combined HRT, there were likely to be 800 extra cases of breast cancer, 700 extra heart attacks, 800 more strokes and 1,800 more blood clots in any year than if they had not taken HRT.

Authors of the Million Women Study report in 2003 estimated that use of HRT by UK women aged 50–64 during the previous decade had caused an extra 20,000 breast cancers, three-quarters of them caused by combined HRT.

An earlier randomized controlled trial, the Heart and Estrogen/ progestin Replacement Study (HERS), had reported in 1998 that combined HRT seemed to do more harm than good. In 2002, a follow-up study called HERS-2 confirmed that HRT did not reduce the number of heart attacks in women in their sixties who already had heart disease. And it increased the risk of gall bladder disease and blood clots.

These independent studies – the Million Women, HERS and WHI – were mainly looking at the long-term effects of HRT on disease after menopause. Critics have said that their results were less relevant to women taking HRT in their forties and early fifties to combat symptoms of the menopause.

However, the Million Women did include some women in their fifties who were still having periods. And there have not yet been any equally large independent studies of younger women taking HRT.

DID MEDICS DO A U-TURN?

The 2007 re-analysis of the WHI study looked at the youngest women, those in their early fifties – closer to the age at which women are most likely to take HRT for symptoms of the menopause. It found their increased heart-disease risk was slightly lower than that of the older women. The women taking oestrogen-only HRT were not at increased risk of breast cancer either.

Media headlines at the time claimed that experts had had to back down on their previous warnings, as the evidence now showed HRT was safe. However, this was not the case.

The re-analysis showed that some HRT risks were slightly lower for certain women, including those taking oestrogen only. However, oestrogen-only HRT increases the risk of womb cancer, so it is not prescribed except for women who have already had hysterectomies.

On heart disease, the re-analysis showed that the increased risk affected older women more, but that the difference in risk between younger and older users was not large enough to be statistically significant.

The increased risk of strokes, blood clots and breast cancer remained valid for all ages. The reanalysis had not found a substantial change in overall risks.

Some supporters now say that HRT poses less of a risk than was revealed by the major studies published in and around 2003. But the general trend at present is to discover fewer benefits and more risks. This is partly just correcting the inflated claims that were made for HRT in the previous decades.

HRT and the drug companies

Sales of HRT products are highly profitable. In 2001, global sales were worth £2,400 million, according to the *British Medical Journal* (*BMJ*).

Many drug trials showing the benefits of HRT have been funded by the manufacturers. Research has shown that studies funded by a manufacturer are much more likely to report favourable results than independent studies of the same drug. Industry-funded studies are also more likely to remain unpublished if their results showed the drug in an unfavourable light.

Meta-analyses – studies looking at the results of numerous other studies in a field – were once considered to be more reliable. But the *BMJ* published a study in 2007 showing that meta-analyses funded by a drug company were more likely to report favourable conclusions.

Also, the results of a study or drug trial may be misleadingly reported in the news, either because the reporter didn't understand them or because a public relations company has put a spin on them. In the USA, for example, the Center for Media and Democracy found in 2006 that science news broadcast by US television stations is sometimes prepared not by journalists but by a PR firm.

Manufacturers have funded a lot of publicity promoting HRT. The influential 1966 book *Forever Feminine*, by gynaecologist Robert Wilson, was revealed in 2002 to have been funded by the drug company Wyeth, which makes the most commonly prescribed HRT drugs. During the past few years, drug companies have run several large PR campaigns through organizations such as HRT Aware, and made large donations to menopause charities.

In addition, manufacturers can influence the doctors who write our prescriptions. Drug companies have been found to sponsor medical education in ways that could bias students towards their products.

Australian research published in 2008, for example, showed that drug companies had selected speakers at seminars which had been advertised as 'independent of industry influence'.

Drug companies knew in the 1990s that HRT could increase the risk of heart disease, but did not make this public, the *BMJ* revealed in 2004. Experts from Oxford University had suggested a link between HRT and heart disease in 1997, but had to go through a lengthy legal process to gain access to drug companies' unpublished research. These eventually turned out to confirm the Oxford findings.

Index

Image credits